Home Nursing for Carers

Home Nursing for Carers

With contributions from Saskia Bos,
Ermengarde de la Houssaye and Wil Visser

Tineke van Bentheim

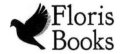

Floris
Books

Translated by Tony Langham and Plym Peters
Illustrations by Walter Krafft and Fiona van Mansvelt

First published in Dutch in 1980 under the title
Zieken thuis by Uitgeverij Vrij Geestesleven, Zeist
First published in English in 1987
Second, revised edition published in 2006
Second printing 2018

British Library CIP Data available
ISBN 978-086315-541-3
Printed by Lightning Source

Contents

Introduction   7

I. Rudolf Steiner's Philosophy and Theory of Nursing

1. Caring, Mediating, Supervising: Three Aspects of Nursing   13

     1.1 Caring 15
     1.2 Mediating 19
     1.3 Supervision 22

2. Rudolf Steiner's View of the Human Being   25

     2.1 The fourfold structure of man 25
     2.2 The threefold structure of man 28
     2.3 Summary 32

3. Plants and the Body   34

II. Treatment

4. The General Care of the Patient   41

     4.1 Furnishing the sick room 41
     4.2 Daily care 44
     4.3 Some nursing aids 54
     4.4 Complications resulting from confinement to bed 56

5. External Treatments   61

     5.1 Outline 61
     5.2 Materials 62
     5.3 Herbal extracts 63
     5.4 General remarks 65

6. Plant Treatments   67

    6.1 Arnica (Arnica montana) *67*
    6.2 Stinging nettle (Urtica urens) *69*
    6.3 Lemons (Citrus media) *74*
    6.4 The marigold (Calendula officinalis) *83*
    6.5 Camomile (Matricaria chamomilla) *85*
    6.6 Horseradish (Cochlearia armoracia) *95*
    6.7 The mustard plant (Sinapis alba *and* nigra) *100*
    6.8 Onion (Allium cepa) *109*

7. Other External Treatments   114

    7.1 Curd cheese (quark) 114
    7.2 Salt water wash 118
    7.3 Baths 120
    7.4 Rubbing the whole body 125
    7.5 Foot-baths 127
    7.6 Poultice 129

III. Birth, Illness and Death

8. Pregnancy and Birth   133

    8.1 Pregnancy 133
    8.2 Birth and confinement 136

9. Sleep   139

10. Sickness and Destiny   144

11. Nursing the Critically and Terminally Ill   147

Remedies to Keep at Home 153
Endnotes 156
Index 157

Introduction

The purpose of this book is to help with the home care and treatment of the sick. We also aim to provide some answers to many questions typically raised by qualified nurses and nursing students, as well as by laymen and other professionals. There often seems to be a problem in arriving at a single form for the various groups. We hope to provide some ideas, both for those caring for the sick at home, as well as for nursing staff looking for a more meaningful approach to their profession and a way of increasing its scope. As regards the form of the book, we believe that practical aspects cannot be considered in isolation from the anthroposophical background — the philosophy established by Rudolf Steiner.

A short résumé of the life and work of Rudolf Steiner is followed by an analysis of nursing practice, stressing the quality of care. Part one concludes with a brief summary of those aspects of anthroposophy necessary to carry out the practical instructions described in the second part. The third part deals with pregnancy and birth, and with the care of the critically ill and the dying.

Rudolf Steiner

Rudolf Steiner was born in Kraljevec on the Austro-Hungarian border in 1861.

While he was studying he met Karl Julius Schröer, a professor of the history of literature, and the meeting was decisive for his development. This friend and mentor introduced him to the work of Goethe. For Steiner, the philosophy expressed in Goethe's work was like a confirmation of his own experiences. He had experienced the spiritual world as a reality since his childhood, and he continued to develop his ways of observing it.

He emphasized the fact that every person has the potential to experience this spiritual world, and in his book, *Knowledge of Higher Worlds*, he explained how it can be achieved. He managed to describe the experiences of his scientific, spiritual investigations in a way that makes it possible for modern man to penetrate the spiritual world with a healthy intellect.

One of the central ideas in anthroposophy is that humankind has developed through many incarnations and has now reached a stage when it can acquire insights into the spiritual world, which exert a new influence on society.

On this basis attempts have been made to apply anthroposophy practically in different areas. In the first place new movements arose in art, literature and the art of movement, known as eurythmy.

The Goetheanum was built in Dornach in Switzerland as an independent college for the sciences of the spirit, and is the international centre for the anthroposophical movement. Many conferences are held there and annual performances take place. There are also laboratories where scientific research is carried out with new methodologies, for example, in the fields of quality control and medical diagnosis.

A number of young theologians turned to Rudolf Steiner to ask whether he could help to breathe new spirit into Christian religious life. This resulted in the foundation of The Christian Community by Friedrich Rittelmeyer.

Rudolf Steiner was asked many questions relating to spiritual reawakening, which eventually led to new developments in the fields of *education* (Steiner or Waldorf schools), *agriculture* (biodynamics), *curative education* (care of the mentally disabled) and *structure of society* (division of the social organism into three parts). His teaching carried an evolution of existing ideas, elaborated with a spiritual dimension.

New ideas were introduced in medicine when the Dutch doctor, Ita Wegman, together with Rudolf Steiner, developed medical doctrine on a profound spiritual basis. A clinic was set up in Arlesheim in Switzerland (now the *Ita Wegman Clinic*). Laboratories were also founded for the preparation of medicines (*Weleda, Wala*).

Ita Wegman took the further initiative of founding a so-called 'therapeuticum' wherever a new practice was set up. This is a place where patients who are not bedridden can, in an environment of peace and harmony, undergo the therapies which form an important part of anthroposphically-based medicine.

There are national anthroposophical societies in a number of countries, and together they form the General Anthroposophical Society, which has its centre in Dornach, Switzerland.

I

Rudolf Steiner's Philosophy
and Theory of Nursing

1. Caring, Mediating, Supervising: Three Aspects of Nursing

Whether done in a nursing home or in a hospital, whether the patients are adults or children, nursing requires knowledge and understanding if it is to be a real 'art.' A knowledge of people in sickness and in health, as well as familiarity with the prescribed treatment and care is essential.

Virginia Henderson describes the unique function of nursing as:

> ... assisting individuals (sick or well) with those activities contributing to health, or its recovery (or to a peaceful death) that they perform unaided when they have the necessary strength, will, or knowledge; nursing also helps individuals carry out prescribed therapy and to be independent of assistance as soon as possible.[1]

Thus the nurse helps with immediate needs like a 'brother' or 'sister,' while the patient is unable to attend to them because of his specific situation.

If a doctor is consulted in the case of illness, he will try to create a picture of the illness on the basis of the case history, the complaints and the symptoms. The therapy is then based on this picture. For it to be as clear and objective as possible the doctor must distance himself. During subsequent consultations the picture may be clarified, or possibly altered. The doctor must rely upon the co-operation and complete honesty of the patient as regards the description of the symptoms and in carrying out the therapy.

Playing at being a doctor oneself is not usually very successful — except for the treatment of common minor complaints and accidents. If there is a basis of mutual trust with one's own general practitioner, the treatment described in this book can usually be discussed and applied without problems.

The doctor and the patient (and possibly the doctor's representative, the nurse) work together closely along the path to recovery. On the basis of the doctor's recommendations, the therapist and patient go step by step together towards a particular goal. Specific possibilities are at the therapist's disposal, for example, physiotherapy, hydrotherapy, eurythmy and a variety of art therapies.

This book is limited to the description of a number of nursing procedures, which can be included amongst the therapeutic possibilities of anthroposophical medicine. They can also be used by parents as procedures for their children, if prescribed by the doctor.

What is meant by the 'art of therapy' in nursing? Nursing is not just caring for the sick, handing out medicine and carrying out the prescribed procedures; it requires a fundamental attitude to help and support a sick person when necessary. The most important therapeutic 'art' consists of being a fellow creature with human understanding of the body, soul and spirit.

In life the body, soul and spirit cannot be divided, though they can be distinguished, and just as this distinction can be made in man, three aspects can also be found in nursing. At any moment one of these three will always be foremost, according to the immediate requirements.

In her previously-mentioned book, *Principles and Practice of Nursing,* Virginia Henderson wrote that the necessity of gauging both the long-term and short-term needs of the individual for physical care, emotional support and rehabilitation makes nursing a 'service of the highest order.'

The word 'patient,' increasingly being replaced by the word 'client,' is retained here as it expresses the need for patience, for allowing time for a process to lead to the acquisition of a new harmony.

1.1 Caring

Caring for the sick takes us into the field of primary bodily needs, such as breathing, regulation of body temperature, eating and drinking, sleeping and waking, adopting a correct posture and moving about. To the extent that the patient is unable to fulfil these needs himself, it is the nurse's task to create the best conditions under the circumstances to keep him alive. At the same time this should be done in such a way that improvement can take place. In this way the care becomes a therapeutic art as a patient gradually regains his independence for the most elementary daily activities.

Caring for a patient should never degenerate into any form of mollycoddling. On the contrary, it is the nurse's task to stimulate independence, helping him to 'incarnate' so that the spiritual essence can reside in his physical body and use it as an instrument.

Although plants do the actual growing, a gardener creates the optimal conditions in his nursery for the growth and healthy development of his plants. And we should do likewise when caring for the sick, always conscious of the fact that the expected healing process originates in the patient himself. It is never possible to force a person to be cured. We can only create the conditions for this to take place, for we are always faced with a particular person and *his* destiny, *his* will to live and *his* chances of recovery. These must always be respected and we must be receptive to what is required at any given moment.

Like the gardener, we are concerned with the quality of the environment; with the four basic elements, earth, water, fire and air. The human environment also includes all the qualities which impinge on the senses, such as light and colour, sound and smell, and so on, as well as specific human qualities, which create a cool atmosphere or a warm atmosphere, and can make the surroundings 'beautiful.'

A first requirement for nursing to become an art is that the techniques for procedures and manipulations are thoroughly controlled, and that the order of the procedures is completely known and imprinted on the consciousness before starting. For example, a procedure should never be interrupted to go and fetch something.

It takes an extremely alert character to observe and empathize with the patient and assess the situation from his point of view. The nurse should notice the empty glass on the bedside table, be aware if the patient is blinded by the light, hear the irritating drip of a leaking tap, hear herself speaking too loudly or too softly, be conscious that she sometimes shuts the door with an aggravating click. There are hundreds of such details to be noted, so that they can be prevented or dealt with, and they are so important that the motto could well be 'Attention to detail.'

(a) The four elements

In 'caring for the environment,' for inner well-being, and for the direct and wider areas of the patient's need, we make use of the elemental qualities — the permanence of *earth*; *water* with its flowing, metamorphosing nature; *air*, with its changing moods, and *heat*, which gives a human quality to everything.

Where the patient's *support system* fails, for instance in the case of a fracture, back pain, loss of equilibrium, support can be provided by splints or plaster, a special mattress, supportive pillow, or possibly a board placed under the mattress, by a stick or a supportive hand below the elbow. With psychological stress a consistent daily routine, and solid, regular meals may help. These provide a sense of security and resistance, which lead to awareness and strengthen self-knowledge. The nurse must be receptive to the patient's needs, so as to know to what extent, and in what form, certainty should be provided.

Water, the liquid element, plays a part in virtually all the processes described in this book, because it is an ideal 'mediator,' and it can take up qualities and substances and then release them. It also plays a part in daily hygiene. Again it is a matter of being observant, seeing how much is required, how *wet* the wash should be. A thorough wash can be marvellously refreshing, for instance, after heavy perspiration. On the other hand, it could also dissolve the last grain of warmth and strength in a dying patient. In such a case one must know how the patient can be refreshed and how to care for his skin.

The drinking requirements of the sick should be given special attention. Too little, or too much, moisture will confuse all the internal relationships. If the patient is unable to drink, or unable to drink enough, the intake of fluids has to take place by other means, for example, through intravenous infusion.

The element of water is inseparably involved in *life*.

Air, which is a primary life requirement as the air we breathe, also has a strong influence on *spiritual life*. Anyone who feels short of breath will soon become fearful; a close atmosphere makes it difficult to stay awake, while the thin air of high altitudes leads to a feeling of light-headedness.

Smells, such as cooking smells, a real stench or a strong perfume, can affect a sick person in a very unpleasant way because he is unable to escape it. However, sometimes the patient feels a need for his 'own' atmosphere and is uncomfortable if the windows are constantly opened to air the room. Moods can hang in the air, just as the weather can be oppressive, threatening or exhilarating. *Humour* is often an invaluable asset in dissolving threatening situations.

Heat is important in the procedures described, as hot and cold stimuli can provoke or inhibit certain processes. It is necessary to discover the correct temperature for every patient individually, by ensuring that he has the right clothing, bed clothes, room temperature, or by providing an extra source of heat or cold.

Heat is also a consideration when the patient is encouraged to be active, or when providing more peace and quiet. Warmth can be expressed in a handshake, a glance, or a meeting between two people. And it really is possible when 'fired' with enthusiasm to become warm inside.

The qualities, which affect the body, also influence the soul. Colours, smells and sound affect physical processes through the more or less conscious experience of the soul.

This brings us to art therapy, as it is possible to use these qualities consciously by bringing colour into the room with flowers, coloured curtains or a tablecloth, or by hanging a painting.

When someone has to be a patient for an indeterminate period (as when bedridden) the senses become more responsive to impressions. These have a profound effect on all the vital processes, as they do on small children. It is no longer possible to shut them out, and the patient becomes 'hypersensitive.' He is also 'hyperaesthetic;' ugly, unpleasant or very strong impressions have much more disturbing effects. On the other hand, there is also the potential for a far more subtle perception of reality, quality and beauty, which can lead to permanently increased sensitivity, if quality is available in every field.

There is a great responsibility for a nurse working in this therapeutic, environmental sense, because all these influences affect the patient's life processes. Nursing can only be a 'service of the highest order' if there is an unbroken intention to help the patient to become independent, and more able to understand himself. A *respect* for this growth and *faith* in the possible recovery of every person form the basic attitude when caring for the sick.

1.2 Mediating

The nurse, as a human being, acts as an intermediary in the nursing function. She (or he) is responsible for continuity of care. One nurse passes the care on to another and together they form a link with the outside world, which is unattainable to the patient himself. They ensure that the relationship with family and friends, nature and the cultural environment, is maintained or re-established.

Just as the god with winged feet, Hermes (Mercury), of classical mythology, was able to act as a messenger to the gods, appearing to gods, humans and in the underworld, so the nurse has the task of maintaining contact with all 'worlds' on the patient's behalf. The nurse is a link, a 'Mercury' figure for the patient. She forges the links for the person entrusted to her care, both in a physical sense (with the outside world) and in a temporal sense (in continuity of care). Besides her empathy with the patient's experiences, pain and needs, she should also be able to understand the viewpoint of other people who are involved, and if necessary, act as an 'interpreter' for these people and the patient.

She should be open to several different spheres, and if these can be assimilated and actually come together in the nurse, this is a true 'heart function.'

The nurse burdens her heart with many problems, weighing them up, assessing their value, and linking them with other situations, of which the inner value is also understood.

It is often extremely difficult to evaluate subtle nuances, because it is often much easier to understand one person rather than another; a common feeling with one brings prejudice in regard to another. The therapeutic art of nursing consists in the nurse seeing *herself as a therapeutic instrument* in carrying out her task. Is it really possible for a person to be a therapeutic instrument, to be 'medicine' for another human being? How does the healing process really come about?

The *substance* of a medicine, for example, is not simply taken from nature; it has been processed in a particular way. Homoeopathically-reduced natural medicines go through a long process of preparation. They are *potentized* by rhythmical processes to improve their quality, while the actual substance is physically present in successively smaller quantities through dilution. It is the inner quality of a particular substance, which is increasingly released in this preparation, and which we 'encounter' when we take this kind of medicine.

A *human* encounter is always essential: the self meets another self. We do not always perceive this when it is happening and are often prejudiced, shutting it out, distracted by external appearances and our own feelings of sympathy or aversion. Nowadays, it is very rare for people to have an essential encounter in a natural and spontaneous way.

A probation is necessary for anyone who wishes to enter the caring profession and become a therapist. An understanding of the self and the emotions, as well as personal self-knowledge and self-control, are prerequisites for the naturalness and tolerance necessary for any essential encounter to take place. Rudolf Steiner advised nurses to concern themselves with the patient's moods or humours, and to use this as an area of research. He considered this to be the real work of nursing. These moods, humours and changeable states of mind (both pleasant and unpleasant) arise when a person has not really got himself under control and is not completely 'present.'

The mood is stronger than the person himself: a familiar phenomenon in cases of sickness or overtiredness, in a crisis, or simply a Monday morning. Every parent, every nurse knows the constant demands, repeated calls or rings for nothing in particular, constant pleas for attention. At that moment the patient cannot be satisfied and does not really wish to be. He may feel very unhappy about his behaviour but simply cannot help acting as he does. Such moods can be infectious! Before you know where you are, you may have answered in the same tone of voice and reacted in similar irritation. Involuntarily you are dancing to the patient's tune. In this situation the nurse is more of a mirror than a therapeutic instrument, and reacts without really paying any heed to what the patient is saying through his expressions of discontent.

To be able to see through all this requires a high degree of self-knowledge, and at the same time a capacity to understand the patient in order to judge the situation from his point of view.

Sometimes an explosive argument or quarrel is a healthy way of clearing the air, and it can give both parties a chance to come to their senses. Nevertheless, it is the task of the nurse to evaluate which 'solution' is necessary, and possible, in any situation.

An almost superhuman strength is necessary to be a 'therapeutic instrument' day after day, in regular contact with a patient. Even as an intermediary, it is only possible to create *conditions*, so that the encounter can have an awakening effect. The first conditions have to be created in ourselves — putting our own soul in order. This frees us to show an *interest* in another person, his pain and fear, his discomfort and insecurity, so that we do actually feel them. This interest, arising between us, can be experienced as an objective force, which opens the way for the patient's recovery. With active interest — our empathy or love (whatever term is used) — we create the conditions for using ourselves as a 'therapeutic instrument.' This forms the basic attitude for the nurse to act as an intermediary.

1.3 Supervision

The supervisory function of the nurse consists of sharing all the patient's ups and downs, day after day. In this sense the term 'brother' or 'sister' is extremely appropriate; the nurse is prepared to share the patient's destiny for a while, to empathize with him, and also to prepare him for what the future will bring. This may simply be a meal, an injection or treatment, a visit, an examination or an operation. But the better prepared the patient is, the better able he his to cope with a possibly unpleasant situation, as a person who is conscious of the self; and the less likely he is to feel uncertain or overwhelmed. Even a joyful event, for example, getting out of bed for the first time, going outside or receiving a visit, can be rather threatening if it has not been properly prepared for. He may not be able to meet the situation and will make all sorts of objections.

However, the worst thing for anyone is to feel that he is no longer seen as a human being, and to start to think of himself as an object or a number.

If consciousness of the self has been weakened by some crisis in the patient's life, or if he has no 'view' of the course of his life, so that he is unable to follow it independently, the nurse can accompany him as a brother or sister, faithful to his essential self, to the person.

An example of this type of supervision is described in the Book of Tobit in the Apocrypha to the Old Testament. The story is set during the period of captivity in Niniveh. Tobit, an aged man, remained faithful to God and the Law, but he grew poor and went blind. He sent his son, Tobias, to recover some money that he had once lent to a friend. Tobias had to make a long journey. He was young and inexperienced and Tobit, therefore, sought a travelling companion for him. Tobias himself found a young man who was prepared to travel. He did not know it was really the angel Raphael, and he greeted him, saying: 'Do you know the way to the land of Media?' The angel answered: 'I know the way, I have often travelled along that road.'

This companion filled Tobias with courage in threatening situations, told him what was going to happen, and gave him instructions about what to do. When Tobias returned with the debt repaid he was able to cure his father's blindness.

The angel, Raphael, knew the way ahead, but also accompanied Tobias on this difficult journey. These are the two sides to supervision: looking ahead and accompanying. As human beings we cannot know the way as well as the angel. However, we can practise reading the map by learning the general laws of life, illness and death.

It can also be extremely rewarding to study biographies, as examples of 'journeys.' Every person goes his own way, with an entirely individual approach to a given situation. An event, which casts one person down, can give strength to another to resist it. For the nurse it is a question of being sensitive to what speaks through the events: the person.

This sensitivity, a looking for possible roads together, is often helpful. Perhaps the new road is not yet visible, but there may be some light in the situation. A sense of *purpose* can become apparent from a survey of the whole life.

We normally live our life with a great lack of awareness: events come towards us, we carry out certain actions, and we only realize in retrospect what the important moments were. Events experienced as setbacks or accidents may be found to have had a very positive effect. This can engender confidence in the purpose of the current situation. It can also give the necessary courage to take hold of it and make the most of it.

Towards the end of life and at the point of death, it becomes increasingly important to accompany the patient step by step on his way, as a brother or sister, neither anticipating nor lagging behind the actual situation.

When nursing dying patients, the care, mediation and supervision increasingly intermingle. Caring for the body and the environment form the supervision, and the anticipatory care to meet future needs is possible through the strength derived from an interest in, or empathy with, another human being. This is the essence, the therapeutic art of nursing in which the nurse is, above all, a fellow human being.

2. Rudolf Steiner's View of the Human Being

To arrive at an understanding of the therapeutic art described in the previous chapter, we should outline the view of man on which it is based. The following is a very brief summary of a subject that is dealt with in detail in other anthroposophical literature.

2.1 The fourfold structure of man

As regards his body, man is one with the surrounding natural world, minerals, plants and animals. It is possible to distinguish the purely *physical* (material) *body,* which man has in common with the *mineral kingdom.* It consists of matter, elements of the material world, and complies with the same laws.

The physical body is permeated by a principle of a different nature, the *body of life* or *etheric body*, which turns the physical body into a living body with form and shape. This is subject to the new and different laws inherent in life which to some extent raise the physical body above physical laws. These laws can also be discerned in *plants*, in their growth and flowering and in their great diversity of form. The life-body can be described as the 'architect.'

In death, the life-body withdraws and the physical body is once again subject to physical laws and loses its form. The living body is not perceptible to the senses, though its effects can be perceived.

In addition, there is a world of impressions and feelings to which man can react with a part of his inner self, known as the *perceiving or sentient soul.* It permeates the physical and ethereal, leads to the development of organs and senses, and is responsible for the possibility of movement. Man has this soul in common with animals, though the latter are much more strongly connected with it, and it actually delimits their behaviour. Animals react directly to stimuli from the outside world, whether they are seeking shelter from thunder, shivering with fright or joyfully hopping up to another animal.

The inner world of animals is comparable to the inner world of humans, though there are some essential differences. We human beings are not completely subjected to the feelings which arise in us; we are able to think and observe them, from a distance. We do not simply experience sympathy or antipathy; our individual soul communicates with everything taking place around us in space and time.

The human soul also has a spiritual strength, which enables it to free itself from the desires of the physical body. Everyone knows these desires, but everyone is also aware of feelings of truth, beauty and goodness, which can be developed and enhanced.

Unlike animals a human being has a core of spirituality and morality, which gives his life purpose and content by forming and guiding it. This divine, spiritual core, which can also be called the Self, makes it possible for him to think and act creatively.

By thinking, we are able to penetrate the essence of plants, animals and colours around us, and in fact any other phenomena of the physical world. Normal brain structure is a prerequisite for this activity, but it is only a prerequisite. With the Self we are able to take our own development in hand and discover profound relationships and backgrounds. We are free to follow a particular developmental path, or to discover the spiritual world.

The individual, our spiritual core, is expressed not only in our posture, facial expression and gestures, but also in our biography, the course of our life. Particular skills or qualities are often ascribed to heredity, but no one who has observed the strange differences, for example, between brothers and sisters, will be wholly satisfied with this explanation. A life cannot simply be explained in terms of coincidence. This will be obvious to anyone with an open mind from the situations in which people find themselves, the tasks that face them, and the encounters with other people that give purpose to life. Of course, heredity governs a part of everyone's life, but the question is how the individual spiritual core, or Self, responds to this, and what effect it has. Anthroposophy shows that this Self endures through different situations, in different eras, with different cultures, and actually develops in the process.

It is the heritage and experience from a previous life, which largely determine our current life and particularly its task. This being so, the main question is how we use the talents with which we are now endowed, and how this affects our destiny. We look at the way in which particular joyful events, disappointments or illnesses are dealt with, rather than at the visible results.

A person can gain strength from an illness or from suffering, and this can have an effect on future life. Very ill people often reveal an impressive strength, which enables them to bear and assimilate a process. Another human being who accompanies the sufferer on his path can be of great help in this.

Thus, the lives of different people contain situations, which are almost impossible to compare. The question to ask is: from what reality shall I give form and content to my life?

In the life, death and resurrection of Christ, a renewing and divine force, leading to the future, was connected with the earth and mankind. Man can be aware of his connection with this strength in the depths of his being, even (and even especially) in conditions of illness.

2.2 The threefold structure of man

Above we gave a brief description of the structure of man in relation to the natural world around him.

However, for anthroposophical medicine it is also important to recognize the basic structure of the body as an expression and an instrument. Recognition of this structure, in three parts, is fundamental.

The human figure can be divided into the head, trunk and limbs. The head is carried by the body and we walk on earth with our legs, while the arms accompany this movement, and remain free to act.

When we examine the function of the head and limbs, it is noticeable how we actively approach the future with the limbs, while the head can peacefully review and consider the past.

The main part of the head is the *nervous/sensory system* where there is virtually no metabolism; the nervous system does not regenerate itself, a dead nerve cell is not replaced. The colours of both the white and grey matter of the brain reveal that this is a place where peace and coldness reign. We have waking consciousness to thank for this; for example, a headache is soothed by cold; for instance, a cool hand, a cold face flannel (face-cloth) or even an ice-pack on the forehead.

In the stomach on the other hand, the constant digestion of matter takes place and cells are continuously regenerated here as metabolism takes place. In digestion the heat of the red blood is needed to process food with great amounts of energy and activity. (A stomach ache can often be relieved with extra heat, for instance a hot water bottle.) We are quite unconscious of all these bodily processes. Movement is characteristic of the *metabolic/limb system* while even the slightest movement of the brain (which floats in cerebro-spinal fluid) will result in concussion. In other words, the principle, the tendency of the nervous/sensory system, is the opposite to that of the digestive/limb system. Neither should become so dominant that it enters the area of the other system, as this can result in disorders.

This polarity between the upper and lower, tranquillity and movement, achieves some equilibrium by means of a third principle of energy, the *rhythmic system,* which is mainly active in the central regions. It acts as an intermediary between the extremes, and harmonizes the two different poles. The movement of the chest is slight, it accompanies the breathing in and out of the lungs. The movement of the heart is in rhythmical relation with this: systole and diastole. As the heart contracts (systole) it reveals the formative principle of the nervous/sensory system, while the expansion (diastole) reveals that of the digestive/limb system.

In general, rhythm is a true central element. Rhythm arises where stillness and movement meet. The process of the upper pole, which has more to do with consciousness, is partially extended in respiration, which can be consciously influenced. The lungs lie at the top and back of the chest cavity. The circulation is related to the heart and cannot be influenced consciously. Constructive strength is passed to all the organs by the warm blood.

A person will only suffer from an illness of the rhythmic area if either the upper or the lower pole is dominant. If the upper pole is dominant, this results in rigid, hardening diseases; when the lower pole is dominant, this results in infections, in the widest sense of the word.

> It is the function of the rhythmical system to ensure
> that neither the building process of metabolism, nor
> the breaking down process of the nervous system
> gains the upper hand, as this must result in illness.[2]

The processes of these two poles, which exist throughout the body should only be dominant within their own fields. In illness they break down barriers and start to dominate in other areas. In addition to the use of medicines, external and art therapies, attempts will always be made to reintroduce rhythm as a factor in the daily life of a patient. Dr L.F.C. Mees said:

> Thus we see that the whole body is divided into these three elements, which are differently arranged in different parts but are so closely related as a whole that the result is harmonious interaction. As long as the rhythmic system is able to continue as a central area between the two polarities, any disturbances of equilibrium can be rectified.[3]

The three principles can also be distinguished in the structure of the skeleton and they are made visible by form. The most noticeable feature of the *head* is its round shape. This is due to the way in which the flat bones (in adults immovably fused together along the seams) enclose the brain and an important proportion of the nerves.

This is also where important sensory organs are situated, including the ears, eyes and nose, with which we perceive the outside world in sounds, colours and smells. In addition, this is where we take in food, which is experienced through taste. The outside world reaches us through these various entrances, and this is how we become conscious of the world. This is where we find the greatest concentration of nervous and sensory processes.

The *limbs*, which consist of hollow bones, radiate to the periphery, starting from a single bone in the upper arm and leg, then two in the lower arm and leg leading to the various small bones in the fingers and toes. The bones are surrounded by tissue and muscle. In contrast with the seams of the skull, the joints allow for a great deal of movement. This is an example of the metabolic/limb system.

In the skeleton of the *trunk*, the twelve pairs of ribs (the upper ribs), which partially enclose the heart and lungs, are fairly fixed like the skull, while the lower ribs (floating ribs) are not attached to the breastbone like limbs. In other words, this is a meeting point of the two principles of quiet and movement. It is also fascinating to see the gradual transition of the three forces in the thirty-two vertebrae. The structure of the thoracic vertebrae, the central group, reveals a harmony between the processes of the upper and lower groups. The rhythmical element is clearly expressed.

The three principles of force recognizable in the external organization of the body, form the basis for the three spiritual forces: thought, feeling and will.

Thought, which is related to consciousness, has a physical basis in the nervous and sensory system. The brain provides the possibility for creating images and concepts, for reviewing past actions, evaluating them or relating them to other actions.

The *will*, which, by contrast, operates entirely unconsciously can focus upon the execution of a simple action, but can also comprise vital drives in us, as a higher, more profound will. Will is based in the metabolic/limb system. We enter the world, facing the as-yet-unknown future with this system.

Between these two there is *feeling*, with which we react directly to the situation at hand: it is concerned with the here and now. We turn white with shock, go red with rage and our heart beats fast with joy. Sometimes we lose our breath with fear or tension. This clearly shows how a psychological event has a direct physical effect on the rhythmic system.

Thus, the three spiritual forces — thought, feeling and will — are related as psychological functions to the anatomical and physiological constitution of man in his entirety. The interwoven character of the various forces derives its special significance from the personality concerned, who gives a particular 'colour' to the organism at his disposal by the development he has gone through.

2.3 Summary

In order to obtain an accurate idea of what happens during illness, we shall summarize these processes briefly as a preparation for the second part.

The *nervous/sensory processes* are concentrated mainly in the upper part of the body, the head. These are the processes which enable man to be conscious of his perceptions. In the head, the brain tissue and the nervous tissue, which is found throughout the body, most cells are unable to regenerate themselves. Thus processes of consciousness seem to operate at the expense of structure, and even depend on breaking-down processes.

The *metabolic/limb system*, which is concentrated mainly in the stomach, in contrast to the digestive organs, is capable of regenerating itself to a significant extent. Its processes are responsible for 'building' the body, and they occur entirely unconsciously.

The *rhythmical system* is situated in the central part. The processes of the upper and lower parts of the body operate there to an equal extent — it is a sort of balanced meeting point. Rhythm is created in which rest and movement alternate.

In the following illustration (a) shows the healthy interaction of the three processes (the shape of the triangle is arbitrary). If this balance is disturbed, the result is illness. As there can be many different causes, the constitutional characteristics of a person influence the nature of the disturbance. Aspects concerned with eating habits, upbringing, age and social circumstances will colour the way in which the disturbance manifests.

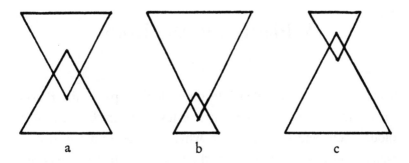

a   b   c

Processes can 'go over the top,' so that, for example, the nervous/sensory processes start to dominate even in the lower half of the body (b), or the lower half starts to dominate in the upper half c. Whether the lower half in (c) really does dominate, or whether the upper half is insufficiently strong and, therefore, ineffective, depends, among other things, on the above-mentioned factors. The ability to recognize these in diagnosis is essential to the therapy used.

The rhythmic system itself cannot be the origin of the illness. However, illnesses can occur in the rhythmic system because the processes of the upper or lower half of the body start to dominate, or are inadequate.

Various external treatments may be applied to diminish processes in the upper half of the body. When the lower half is dominant above it is also possible to stimulate the metabolic limb processes by applying hot compresses.

The second part of this book contains a number of guidelines for these forms of treatment.

3. Plants and the Body

Plants can also be divided into three distinct parts: the *flower*, which can be striking to a greater or lesser extent because of its colour, scent and size; the *leaf*, which can be found in diverse shapes; and finally, the *roots* of the plant, which are largely hidden below the earth.

Some plants are remarkable for their extensive root system, while they have an unremarkable flower, for example, the horseradish, while others, such as camomile, have an abundance of flowers. There are also plants, such as the stinging nettle, which have many leaves and relatively few, small flowers and roots. Other plants are remarkable for their needle-shaped leaves.

Obviously, there are many other plants with almost perfect harmony in the development of leaves, flowers and roots. Examples of these include the rose, the buttercup and the daisy.

Apart from these visible features, there are others, such as scent, etheric oil, and seed formation (etheric oil is a non-greasy, usually volatile, vegetable oil).

Some plants, and families of plants, have a specific affinity to heat, sunlight and other forces operating in nature. This can be expressed in different parts of the plant and in different ways, for example in a strongly-scented root, in a leaf containing small 'pearls' of etheric oil, or in a flower, which wilts quickly and immediately goes to seed. This seed may also contain a lot of oil and have a strong scent.

The phenomena mentioned above suggest that all plants or families of plants have a specific appearance, or even that they all seem to have a one-sided character. This is a result of their strong affinity with one of the three force principles, which operate in nature or the world of plants.

Thus, the horseradish plant is related to the forces, which form a strong root. It contains many important substances (see Section 6.6). In the carob plant the relationship with the quality of heat is a striking feature, and this is shown in that it produces a large amount of etheric oil in the leaf, as well as a beautiful flower.

These examples show that the one-sided nature of plants is also their strength. An extensive root, flower or leaf development, expressing the operative force, produces an operating 'example' for the human organism.

What happens in the roots and the leaves? What has the flower got to tell us?

It is well-known that when the *roots* of a plant are damaged, the leaves, and soon after, the flower, begin to wilt. When plants are fertilized they do a lot of growing in a short time. Thus the roots enable the plant to take in water and nutrients. In addition, the plant perceives the environment, the composition of the soil, through its roots. The roots are only able to perform this function if they are largely underground, in a dark and rather cool environment.

Green chlorophyll is formed in the *leaves* of the plant, and this makes it possible to exchange oxygen and carbon dioxide. By day the plant takes in carbon dioxide and releases oxygen through the leaf; at night, the process is reversed. The essential elements for this 'respiratory' process are air, light and space.

The plant arrives at a final stage when it *flowers*. When this is achieved, the essential contact with the animal kingdom is made. The contact with butterflies and insects is an important link for the fertilization of many flowers. When the flower has wilted and the seed has been formed, there is a possibility of renewed life. The flower can bloom and the seed can flower only if the conditions are sufficiently warm.

Thus, we see that there are three processes, which form the foundation for the life of plants: perception, respiration and regeneration. The same processes were described in man (Section 2.2). As described for plants they appear reversed in humans. Man perceives with his nervous/sensory system, centred in the upper half of his body, while plants achieve their form of perception in the lower regions, through the roots. Because man also has a soul and a spiritual core, the Self, he is capable of self-consciousness by means of his faculty of perception. Perceptive processes can only take place if he is at rest and cool.

There is a constant exchange in the rhythmic system, which is centred in the chest cavity (particularly in the heart and lungs). Unlike plants, man breathes in oxygen and breathes out carbon dioxide by day.

Man is capable of growth, reproduction and physical action through the metabolic/limb system, which is centred in the organs of the stomach and limbs. Warm blood is essential for activity, just as the warm sun is essential for flowers to bloom and bear seed.

Imagine that the nervous/sensory processes have been weakened in a person, making his capacity for thought and perception more difficult because they cannot operate in the necessary restful and cool conditions. The theory outlined above shows how by administering a plant with a one-sided nature visibly centred in the root, a healthier balance may be induced. Plants, whose strength and one-sided nature lie in the leaf, will influence man's rhythmic system, and flowers and seeds will affect the metabolic/limb system.

In practice, the processes are far more complicated than as described above. The physician's skill is required to find out what has gone wrong. According to his diagnosis, he will determine the way in which the plant is prepared and administered. Thus,

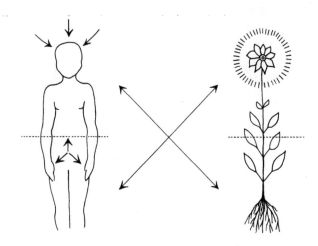

➤ *Human beings perceive through their nervous/sensory system centred in the head, while plants take in their surroundings through the roots. Human growth, reproduction and action is centred in the metabolic/limb system, while in plants it is centred in the blossom and fruit.*

one could imagine that a preparation from a root might be given to influence nervous/sensory processes also taking place in the region of the metabolic/limb system.

However, effectiveness will depend on the way in which the preparation is prepared and administered.

II

Treatment

In this part an attempt is made to forge a link between theoretical and practical considerations.

The previous part described how three principles operate, beginning with the human form. The effect of these three principles (nervous/sensory, respiratory/circulation and metabolic/limb system) on the human organism can be ascertained from careful observation. In a sick person there has been a shift within these functions; an increase or decrease of one of the principles is often the visible consequence of this. However, it is often difficult to observe and express exactly what is the matter. Which principle is dominant and which process has become weaker as a result?

It can be informative to list a number of symptoms of an illness to learn to distinguish various processes which might be disturbed in the entire picture. When this has become clear, it will be possible to give more effective treatment.

After a study of the general care of the patient and the arrangement and furnishing of the sick room, a chapter on external treatments includes descriptions of the plants used in these treatments. By outlining their properties the essential aspect of each plant can be discovered.

4. The General Care of the Patient

In order to treat a sick person at home, a few conditions must be met both for the person doing the nursing, and for the patient and the environment.

We assume that the patient has his own room, or at least a separate room. There certainly are situations where it might be preferable to nurse the patient in the living room so that he is constantly involved in family life, but for seriously ill patients this is not advisable. Obviously, it is out of the question to nurse a patient suffering from a contagious disease in the living room. Apart from these factors, and depending on the general and social circumstances, the doctor, or the person nursing the patient, could still decide to care for him in his own room.

4.1 Furnishing the sick room

For the patient it is best if the *bed* can be placed where daylight enters from the side. It is tiring to look into the light. For the nurse it is best if the bed is away from the wall on three sides. A *bedside table* or cabinet should be placed so that it is easily within the patient's reach. Often it is placed neatly next to the bed at pillow height. However, this arrangement is actually very inconvenient for the patient, as it means that he has to reach diagonally behind him. Push the bedside table slightly forwards so that everything the patient needs is really just within reach.

A bedside table full of flowers, photographs and other knick-knacks is very impractical as it has to be cleared away for every treatment, meal and so on. If the patient likes to have his things around him, it is best to place another table or cabinet on the other side of the bed. Another possibility is a bed table.

There are a number of things, which do have a place on the bedside table, such as a glass of water. The intake of fluids is an important requirement and the glass should be kept full of water or some other refreshing drink. A lid should be placed on the glass to keep out dust.

For a child it is important to have a doll or other familiar toy by his side.

A small bunch of flowers in the room can be effective. However, strongly-scented flowers right next to the bed can be disturbing, and it is better if they are placed elsewhere in the room. Sometimes, the patient can suddenly complain of an itch, a rash or watery eyes. This could be due to an allergy or over-sensitivity to a particular flower or plant. For example, a number of people are very sensitive to primulas, lilies of the valley, ox eye daisies and chrysanthemums. It is a good idea to remove all flowers and plants from the sick room at night.

A note-pad is very useful, and part of the attention to detail that is so important is to make sure that there is also a pen or pencil.

The patient should certainly have a bell or a stick at hand, or some other way of making himself heard when he needs assistance.

The first chapter described how the senses in a sick person become increasingly sensitive to impressions. In the sick room, *pictures* on the wall are very important and can have a positive or a negative effect. This is particularly noticeable in bedridden patients or patients who have a fever. The often rather illusory representations on posters become increasingly intrusive and start 'to speak their own language' in a negative way. This can result in extremely unpleasant experiences; the patient's eyes are constantly drawn to the picture, and because he is ill, he is unable to shut out this effect. In general, he will not express these feelings, and it is therefore up to the person nursing him to take into account what pictures are on the wall. If you really try to put yourself in the patient's place, you may decide to change the picture for another, after talking to him. This can again be replaced with another after a while. Because the senses become over-sensitive, the patient will experience the impressions of colours and images more intensely. By ensuring that these impressions of colours and images are changed, it is possible to 'feed' the patient's subtle sense of quality.

Time is an important factor for anyone who is ill. We will not go into ways of passing the time here, as this is an individual matter and depends on the patient, his illness, his capabilities and limitations. After a while, a creative approach is required to think of the right activities.

Usually the ticking of an alarm clock on the bedside table can easily be heard by the patient — too easily, after a while — and it can become irritating. This can be remedied by placing the alarm clock on a thick piece of material or felt. Then a glass, bell-jar or transparent bowl can be placed over the clock, and this will considerably reduce the noise.

Other noises, which may be very irritating for the patient, include dripping taps or squeaking and banging doors. In most cases this can easily be dealt with, for example, by tying a piece of material round the tap, a towel around the doorknobs, or putting a spot of oil on the hinges. This kind of simple attention can contribute to the patient's peace of mind.

There should be enough *electric light* in the patient's room, though it must not be too strong or shining in his eyes. It is dangerous, and a fire hazard, to tie a piece of material around a light that is too bright. Night-lights are available, which give a very gentle light and can be plugged straight into the socket. This can be useful specially for sick children.

The *temperature* of the room will vary from 20–22 C (68–72 F) depending on the need of the patient. In general, elderly patients and sick people with little resistance require a slightly warmer environment.

It is important for the sickroom to be regularly *ventilated*, for example, with a small window or open door, but watch out for damp.

Finally, there should be a wastepaper basket near the bed, or possibly a paper or plastic bag hanging on the bed.

4.2 Daily care

Meals, usually an important feature in the patient's daily life, are often preceded by taking medicines.

It is important to ensure that meals are always tastefully arranged and served. In general patients will have a poor appetite compared with healthy people and, therefore, smaller amounts of food in various different dishes will be more attractive than a large plate of bubble and squeak.

It is good for the patient to eat his meal in peace, when the room has been cleared and he has emptied his bladder. The bed-side table or cabinet can be attractively laid and a napkin must not be forgotten.

Depending on the patient's illness or handicap, he may need some help with feeding or even have to be fed. This is difficult for many people to accept. Often a patient will be able to help himself with specially adapted crockery or cutlery. For example, special drinking bowls are available from chemists for patients who find it difficult to co-ordinate their movements, or who have to lie flat on their backs. Another solution is to use flexible straws. If the patient is only able to consume a hot meal very slowly it is advisable to use a plate, which can be kept hot with hot water.

44

As much variety as possible in the composition of the menu will stimulate both the appetite and the digestive processes. However, if the patient is on a restricted diet this important variety can be rather a problem. Many health food shops will offer interesting suggestions, or they may know of a dietician whom you can contact.

If a patient is feverish, it is important to make sure he has enough to drink. The body constantly loses more fluid through the skin and in respiration as a result of the increased metabolic activity. It is a good idea to drink small quantities at regular intervals, whether fresh fruit juice, tea or barley water (see end of Section 5.3) to compensate for the salt loss resulting from perspiration.

Milk and milk products should certainly be avoided if the patient is feverish, as well as other foods rich in protein, such as eggs, meat, beans and grains. It is only when the body temperature is back to normal (37°C, 98.6°F) and remains stable, that proteins can gradually be reintroduced.

When the patient has a temperature, it is best to give him (in addition to various fluids) apple purée (which tastes fresh and doesn't leave a slimy taste in the mouth), fruit salad and easily digestible raw vegetables. For a hot meal, cooked greens are easily digested.

It is important to take particular care of the patient's *mouth* when he has a fever. Apart from brushing the teeth, it is a good idea to rinse his mouth regularly (for example, with a mouthwash or half a glass of water with a few drops of lemon juice in it) in order to prevent ulcers in the mucous membrane of the mouth, or rapid decaying of the teeth. The patient will also benefit from having his lips regularly treated with lip salve, as they dry out very quickly.

Make sure that despite his small food intake, the patient has regular bowel movements.

The patient will need to *rest*, especially after his midday meal. Draw the curtains, and when he is well tucked up, the window can be opened to air the room.

For patients who have difficulty in sleeping at night, an afternoon nap is particularly welcome. Unlike heavy sleepers they will be more inclined to take forty winks at intervals during the day. However, this should be prevented as far as possible or the day may be turned into night; a reversal that will certainly not advance the patient's recovery. Try to find a good balance between day and night by providing enough distractions during the day, with a period of rest after the midday meal.

This is also important for those who do sleep well. Everyone needs to be alone and undisturbed at some time during the day.

For people who find it difficult to fall asleep, a mug of warm (aniseed-flavoured) milk or a cup of herb tea (camomile, mallow or lime blossom) can help. It is not advisable for the patient to read the newspaper or any exciting literature in the evening. This may have a disquieting effect for a long time in the night. On the other hand, reading a fairy-tale can be conducive to sleep.

The passing of urine can change in a sick person, both as regards frequency and quantity. Urination often decreases with a fever because a lot of fluid is lost in other ways, like perspiration. The urine is usually more concentrated and darker in colour. If the quantity and frequency of urination decreases too much, and the small quantities of urine are extremely concentrated, it is possible that the patient is drinking too little. If this is not the case, there may be other reasons, and it is advisable to consult the doctor.

There may also be difficulty in moving the bowels because of reduced mobility. The functioning of the intestines is usually slowed down. This can be largely avoided by proper feeding, for instance a diet rich in cellulose (unless the doctor has prescribed otherwise) consisting, for example, of apples, oranges, brown bread, rye bread and grains such as wheat, barley and brown rice. In addition, soaked prunes, bran and linseed in yoghurt (linseed is the seed of the flax plant) are very good.

Bulking agents or laxatives may be used after consulting the doctor. Similarly, Clairo tea, and tea prepared from senna pods, will stimulate peristalsis in the intestines, but the first time they are taken they can produce considerable cramp. This can be painful and is sometimes accompanied by other symptoms, such as palpitations and dizzy spells, and the patient may even faint. This is by no means uncommon and, therefore, laxative tea should be brewed very weakly and tablets should only be taken in small doses. Be especially careful the first few times.

As an aid to the movement of the bowels, keep a margin of two or three days, depending on the patient's normal pattern. If the measures that have been taken fail, and the patient has not had a bowel movement for four or five days, the doctor should be consulted. It might be helpful to replace the bedpan with a commode if possible.

If the patient is suffering from diarrhoea, he should certainly not have a diet rich in cellulose. He should fast and have no more than dry rusks with weak tea or white rice with medicinal bilberry juice, or if the diarrhoea is very bad, just rice water for two or three days. Make sure he takes enough fluid (possibly a thin broth), as a great deal of fluid is lost through diarrhoea.

In the case of repeated vomiting, it is best not to give the patient any solid food for at least twenty-four hours. He should only drink small quantities. (Make sure his head is held to the side to prevent the vomit going down his windpipe, and then rinse out the mouth or give it a wash.)

It is important to ensure absolute hygiene, especially when looking after patients who have diarrhoea or are sick. This means washing the hands thoroughly and regularly, and changing the bed frequently. The toilet should be cleaned at least once a day, as should the door-handles, the handle for flushing the toilet and the taps.

Furthermore, great care should be taken with the crockery and cutlery that has been used. First rinse with boiling (soda) water. The vegetables to be prepared should be rinsed a number of times and any leftovers should be thrown away. Infections can be passed on to other people in many different ways. Diarrhoea can be caused by food that is already infected or spoiled. This risk is particularly prevalent in the summer (paratyphoid).

(a) Giving a bedpan

Shut the windows, and if necessary, the curtains, and wash your hands. The bedpan is placed on a stool next to the bed; also get a towel ready, some toilet paper and a jug or bottle with lukewarm water. Pull back the covers as far as the patient's knees, and when he raises himself slightly you can slide the towel beneath his buttocks. Now place the lid of the bedpan on the stool, and supporting the patient with your hand under his legs, slide the bedpan beneath his buttocks with the other hand. If possible the patient should sit up, supported by his pillows. Make sure his legs are spread and slightly drawn up. Cover him with a sheet. Female patients can be rinsed with some lukewarm water from a jug or bottle. After urinating, the patient raises himself slightly again while his legs are supported and the bedpan is removed. Put the lid on the bedpan. Using the towel, on which the patient is lying, dry him off to prevent infections. The under-sheet is pulled taut and the patient is covered up. The cushions are plumped and turned round.

When the bedpan is emptied, the urine should be checked. If it is noticeably abnormal, pour a small amount in a clean jam-jar so that it can be examined by the doctor.

To clean the bedpan it is best to keep a large jug or bottle of water with soda and a brush in the toilet. The edge should be dried with toilet paper.

Some people find it difficult to pass water when using a bedpan. You can help by supporting the patient in a more upright position (if this is possible and not forbidden by the doctor), by running the tap, giving the patient some water and warming the edge of the bedpan first by rinsing it with warm water. Another possibility is to place a hot water bottle on the patient's bladder. The hot water bottle should be one third full, the air expressed and the tap screwed on tightly. When this has been done, cover the patient with the sheet and leave the room for a moment. He will usually find it easier to urinate in these conditions.

When the patient has moved his bowels, first prepare the washing bowl, flannel and soap. While you remove the bedpan, place it on the stool and cover with a lid, and ask the patient to move onto his side. Wipe the anus with toilet paper and then wash. When the bedpan is emptied, examine the contents for any abnormalities, clear up and finally wash your hands thoroughly. If the stools are abnormal (blood, worms etc.) some can be stored in a jar with a piece of card, stiff paper, plastic, wooden stick, disposable spoon or spatula.

If it is possible and the doctor has not forbidden it, it is obviously a good idea for the patient to go to the toilet himself. Make sure he is wearing slippers and a dressing gown, and do not forget to close the toilet window. However, if it is difficult for the patient to go to the toilet, even though he is able to leave the bed, it is possible to use a commode.

(b) Administering a urine bottle

Shut the windows and, if necessary, the curtains, and wash your hands. The urine bottle is placed on a stool next to the bed. In most cases male patients are able to use it themselves. Give it to the patient and cover him up with a sheet. Emptying and cleaning the urine bottle is done in the same way as described above.

NOTE: Because of the danger of infection, neither the urine bottle nor the bedpan should ever be placed on the floor. In fact, nothing that is put in the bed should ever be left on the floor.

(c) Incontinence

If the patient is incontinent, that is, unable to control urination or bowel movements, it is possible to use absorbent pads, which are available from chemists. Change immediately when these are wet or soiled, and also wash the patient to prevent rashes and bedsores (see Section 4.4 (a)). If the incontinence of urine only occurs when the patient coughs or sneezes, female patients will only need a sanitary towel.

(d) Taking the patient's temperature

Patients who have a changeable body temperature should have their temperature taken first thing in the morning. It is best to take the temperature with a rectal thermometer. The patient lies on his side with his knees slightly drawn up. Rinse the thermometer with cold water, shake it vigorously a few times and check that the mercury level is below 35°C (95°). Put a little vaseline on the end of the thermometer and check that it is intact.

If the patient is unable to insert and hold the thermometer himself, place the point up to the mercury in the rectum. Hold the thermometer, cover the patient with the bedclothes and place your other hand on his hip to prevent any sudden movements which could break the thermometer. After three minutes read off the body temperature and make a note of it on a list. If necessary, repeat the process after the afternoon nap and in the evening before the patient goes to sleep.

After rinsing the thermometer, rinse it again with cold water, wipe with cotton wool soaked in alcohol (70 percent) and shake out.

If it is not possible to take the patient's temperature in the rectum, for example, if he suffers from piles, it can be taken under the armpit. This should first be dried with a towel. The end of the thermometer is placed in the armpit and the patient presses his arm against his side. The other arm is placed diagonally across the chest with the hand on the upper arm in order to keep the thermometer in place. Using this method it takes about five minutes to obtain the temperature. An egg timer can be used. If you make a note of the temperature, also note how it was taken. This method of taking it gives 0.5°C (five lines), 0.9°F, lower than a rectal measurement.

NOTE: The patient's temperature should only be taken when he is resting, and not directly after a visit or getting up, but only half an hour later.

(e) Washing the patient

Clear the bedside table and prepare: a glass of water, toothbrush and toothpaste, possibly a mouthwash, a small, empty bowl, a bowl or bucket of warm water, soap, flannel and towels, also a comb, skin care preparations such as cream and talc, clean underwear and pyjamas (if possible, warmed). Meanwhile, give the patient the bedpan. The windows and if necessary the curtains, should be shut and the temperature in the room should be comfortable. First wash your hands.

If the patient is unable to sit up while he is washed, proceed as follows. Place the towel over the top half of the body and brush the patient's teeth, keeping the head to one side to prevent choking. Rinse and let him spit into the bowl.

Next the patient bares his top (or is helped to do so). If he has a paralyzed or painful arm, slide his pyjama top over the good arm. If both are painful, slide the top up along the back to his neck, and if he then puts his chin on his chest, the top can be pulled over his head and off.

If possible, the patient should wash his face and hands himself. Then wash small areas of the upper half of the body with a relaxed hand, using very little soap and making sure that the patient does not get too cold. The soap should be thoroughly removed. Then dry carefully, taking particular care with folds in the skin.

For skin care use a tonic, rubbed into the skin sparingly with a warm hand, avoiding any with a sticky sensation. Sore elbows can also be treated, but if they are very red and irritated, medicinal ointments have a soothing effect. For the folds of the skin, which are particularly prone to sores, becoming red and moist, use a little talc and then rub out thoroughly.

Put on pyjamas. If necessary, pull on the painful or paralysed sleeve first, then the good side. If the patient is afflicted on both sides, proceed as follows: place the pyjamas, unbuttoned, in front of the patient with the seam of the back under the chin. First put both arms into the sleeves, then gather the top from the hem to the collar, and while the patient's chin is on his chest pass it over his head and pull it down his back.

Throw away the water and fill the bowl again. Use another towel for the legs. Loosen the bedclothes at the foot of the bed and fold back to just above the knees so that you can wash the legs. Rub the heels firmly with skin tonic or soothing ointment. Then use another bowl of clean water and bare the lower half of the body. Place the towel beneath the patient's buttocks. Wash the front from the navel to just above the knees; rinse and dry. For female patients, wash from the top down to prevent infections from the urinary tracts. The patient then turns on his side; wash the buttocks and one hip and finally the anal sphincter from the front to the back. Dry thoroughly. The patient should turn around so that you can wash the other hip.

The buttocks often become very sensitive and red after a prolonged confinement to bed. They can be rubbed with skin tonic or soothing ointment. Use a little talcum powder in the groin, folds of the stomach and anal sphincter, and rub thoroughly so that it cannot go grainy and achieve the opposite of the desired effect. Pull on the patient's pyjama trousers and cover him up.

Finally, place the towel for the upper half of the body over the patient's shoulders, and comb his hair.

Clear away everything that was used for washing the patient.

(f) Making the bed

If possible, the patient should get out of bed to stimulate the circulation of the blood. However, if this is not possible, or against doctor's orders, the clean linen you need should first be placed ready, on the radiator if it is cold. Then place the blankets or duvet on a chair at the foot of the bed and cover the patient with the top sheet.

The patient turns onto his side, lying as near as possible to the edge of the bed. The pillows are removed, apart from one, which is left to prevent him knocking against the hard edge of the bed; if necessary, someone else can help to support the patient. Wipe away crumbs and dust, pull the lower sheet smooth and tuck in firmly.

If the under-sheet needs changing, fold or roll up the dirty sheet behind the patient's back. The clean sheet can now be placed on half of the bed. The patient then turns over (or is turned) on his other side, over the dirty sheet towards the clean one. From the other side of the bed, first remove the dirty linen, pull the clean sheet towards you and tuck it in.

If necessary, change the pillowcase, plump the pillows and rearrange them.

When the bedclothes have been tucked in at the foot of the bed, the blankets are loosened so that the toes have some room to move. The rest of the room is tidied up, and you can wash your hands. Depending on the situation, the whole room can be thoroughly cleaned.

It is important to air the room at least for a little while, if possible by opening a window. The patient should be warmly tucked up, especially his shoulders. He can breathe in and out deeply in the fresh air a number of times. However, it may be impossible to air the room in this direct manner. It can then be aired by leaving the door open and opening a window somewhere else. It is still important to cover the patient up warmly.

It is advisable to make sure that the sickroom is tidy and cosy during the morning. Look after the flowers, change the tablecloth if necessary, and hang another picture on the wall.

Check again that everything is right: a glass of fresh water with a cover, handkerchief, note-pad and pen, something to do, a book (and glasses), own wastepaper basket close at hand, bedside table moved forward. Do not forget the bell or the stick, and make sure a sick child has his doll, security blanket or teddy bear.

4.3 Some nursing aids

Most of the articles mentioned here can be obtained from chemists or specialist shops, or even borrowed or rented from voluntary organizations. In Britain they are available at occupational therapy centres or from your local health centre through the district nurse or general practitioner.

BLOCKS to raise the bed. These are used in cases of long-term illness to spare the nurse's back.

BED PULL. This is attached to the head of the bed. The patient can pull himself up by the handle so that his buttocks are raised from the lower sheet. This is convenient when using the bedpan, for washing, rubbing the buttocks with ointment and straightening the bottom sheet.

A BED CRADLE is used if the body or parts of the body need to be relieved from the weight of the blankets. It is important to ensure that the patient is sufficiently warm; if the arch is placed over a paralyzed leg, the patient himself will not be aware of the temperature of his leg. A child's woollen blanket can be placed over both legs, or a woollen blanket across the arch, tucked in on three sides. With paralysed patients *never* use a hot water bottle as the patient will not feel it and will therefore not be able to say if the bottle is too hot, which could result in scalding.

A FOOT REST keeps the patient's feet in a comfortable position and prevents foot drop.

A BACK REST is for nursing patients in a seated or semi-seated position.

BED TABLE. This slides over the patient's bed and has an adjustable surface.

COMMODE. If the toilet is on another floor, or the patient is
unable to get there, a commode in the room can be very
useful; if possible, used with a screen for privacy.

RUBBER SHEET. This is placed across the under-sheet and
then covered with another sheet folded double, which
should reach from just below the pillow to just below the
knees, though the patient should not be made uncomfortable by the hem. In this way the doubled sheet can easily
be changed and the under-sheet stays dry. If the patient
has sensitive skin, a flannel sheet can be put on top.

A SHEEPSKIN FLEECE can be used under the patient to prevent
bedsores. There are special instructions for cleaning
them and information should be sought when one is
obtained.

4.4 Complications resulting from confinement to bed

(a) Decubitus ulcers (bedsores)

In cases of long-term illness the general circulation is poor,
and as a result of lying in the same position for a long time
the pressure on the skin is great. The pressure points are sensitive and quickly become painful and red. The skin may even
break. The points, which are especially sensitive to bedsores,
are those where the bone is just below the surface of the skin,
such as the outer ear, the spinal column, shoulders, elbows,
buttocks, hips, knees, heels and ankles. In addition, patients
with poor circulation (heart or lung disorders), diabetics, para-
plegics, the chronically ill and elderly patients, are particularly
prone to bedsores.

SOME MEASURES FOR THE PREVENTION OF BEDSORES:

A GOOD DIET: alternately rich in vitamins and protein (except during fever), and of good quality.

MOVEMENT: the patient should get out of bed now and then if he is able to and permitted; bedridden patients may lie on their side, back and stomach (at regular intervals and after particular activities).

A SMOOTH, DRY UNDER-SHEET: Make sure that at the sensitive points there are as few layers of material as possible between the skin and the sheet. It is therefore inadvisable to wear pyjama trousers as well as underpants, as they can easily fold, rubbing against the skin.

GOOD SKIN CARE: Use very little soap when washing the patient, and dry thoroughly. It is possible to prevent sores and stimulate the circulation by using a hair dryer blowing hot and cold air alternately. Also rub the skin regularly with small amounts of skin tonic or soothing ointment. The circulation is also stimulated by this rubbing action.

A SHEEP'S FLEECE makes a soft layer. However, this only works if the skin is in direct contact with the fleece; therefore no pyjama trousers should be worn. If the patient finds this unpleasant, a towel can be placed over his thighs and stomach, or he can wear a long nightshirt cut open at the back from the hem to the waist.

If none of these measures is sufficient to prevent pain and redness, consult the doctor. Once there is an open sore, it is very painful for the patient, and intensive treatment is required for the wound to heal.

(b) Contractures

Contractures are particularly common in the joints of the limbs and result from long-term restricted movement, for example, in diseases such as rheumatism and multiple sclerosis. The limbs are permanently fixed in one position. Drop foot is a well-known example, but contractures can also arise in the knees, ankles, hips and elbows.

CONTRACTURES CAN BE PREVENTED BY:

— Making the patient *walk* if this is permitted, and placing him in different positions in bed, for example, ensuring that he lies flat on his back, with only one pillow, both during his afternoon nap and at night.
— Getting the patient out of bed from time to time (after consultation with the doctor or physiotherapist) and turning the ankles and wrists, *bending and stretching* the knees and elbows, tensing and relaxing the muscles, sitting up and lying down.
— Making sure that the *bedclothes* do not weigh too heavily on the patient, and possibly using a blanket arch or down duvet.

(c) Pneumonia

A patient who is bedridden for a long time will often start to breathe very superficially. As a result, their lung function deteriorates and the risk of pneumonia increases. It is, therefore, important to ensure that the patient takes a few deep breaths in and out a few times a day, for example, before and after every meal, while the room is being aired, during physical exercise, when using the bedpan and before going to sleep.

(d) Thrombosis

This can be a serious complication resulting from confinement to bed. If one or both legs are painful, or if the patient complains of cramps in his calves, the possibility of this complication should be borne in mind, and the doctor should be warned immediately. If the patient does not feel any pain, but the leg feels warm and is rather red and swollen, this can indicate the same thing. Often this is accompanied by a slightly raised temperature. Under no circumstances should the patient leave his bed.

(e) Urine retention

Patients who have to be nursed lying on their back often have difficulty emptying the bladder completely. This increases the chances of a urinary tract infection.

(f) Mobilization

The above warnings have shown how important it is for the patient to move around by getting out of bed from time to time, having a wash or going to the toilet. In addition, it is very important to sit up for a while, now and again.

Nevertheless, it may be necessary to stay in bed for a while. When a patient can get up for a few minutes after being confined to bed for a long time, it is best to give some support. Light-headedness and a shaky feeling in the legs are familiar to everyone.

For this reason, it is a good idea for the patient to sit up in bed first (possibly even a few times) and only try to take a few steps the next day. (Are the windows shut, and is the room nice and warm?) Meanwhile, place a chair with armrests next to the bed and help the patient to put on his dressing gown and slippers (which should have some grip). Support him, placing one foot across and in front of his feet when helping him out of bed. Do the same when he gets back into bed to prevent him from slipping. After a few steps the patient sits down on the chair next to the bed. In this sort of situation, as in many others, it is not a good idea to have small rugs scattered on the floor, as the danger of sliding is too great.

When the patient sits by the bed for the first time after a long period in bed, it is necessary to stay in the room, as it is quite possible that he might suddenly feel unwell.

If he faints unexpectedly, lift him up under the armpits and place him in a horizontal position, if necessary on the floor. Cover him with a blanket to prevent cold. He will probably recover after a moment and should be helped back into bed, possibly with the aid of another person.

5. External Treatments

5.1 Outline

Anthroposophical medicine has many different methods for external (topical) treatments. We shall describe a few of these here:

A COMPRESS is a damp preparation applied to a particular part of the body. It can be hot, warm or cold.

A BODY COMPRESS is also damp. However, this is applied around a part of the body.

A MASSAGE, for example, with skin tonic or oil, can be a localized or an all-over method of treatment. It is always followed by wrapping the patient up well or swaddling him, to stimulate a heat reaction.

A BATH is a treatment for the whole body and, with a few exceptions, is also followed by swaddling. Foot-baths, hip-baths and arm-baths are treatments for specific parts of the body.

A WASH is a total treatment and can sometimes be followed by swaddling.

A POULTICE is a localized application given on or around a particular part of the body.

5.2 Materials

The materials used for compresses and poultices are always made of a natural fibre, such as wool, silk, cotton, linen and flannel. No nylon or acrylic fabrics should be used, or any materials containing these artificial fibres. No taffeta, plastic or hospital linen should be used either.

Synthetic fibres are impermeable, and allow little or no air to pass through them. This means that the skin starts to perspire in an unnatural way, and cannot breathe. This form of fluid excretion is prevented in the external methods of treatment used in anthroposophical medicine (with a few exceptions).

By breathing in, man forms a physiological link with the outside world; when he breathes out, the outside world is linked to him — an interaction between man and the world outside him is created in this way. The term 'breathing process' is used in a metaphorical sense when we refer to the alternating movement between the inside and the outside world.

With materials, which do not counteract this process in the external treatments, 'breathing' can take place between the external curative quality of a substance administered to the body and the body's reaction to it. This breathing process can also be described in terms of question and answer; the questions usually come from outside, the answer follows from within. The skin is the most important organ in this activity.

It depends on the illness and its effects, as well as on the nature of the person concerned, whether the organism is capable of 'answering' the question. In some cases the answer is given only when the question has been repeated a few times; sometimes the organism first needs help to understand it before being able to give an adequate answer.

It should be remembered that what happens between the 'asking of the question' and the 'giving of the answer' cannot be described in words. In order to provide effective treatment the doctor and the therapist must constantly reconsider and attempt to create a mental picture of which processes have become disturbed. It is only when this has been established that the correct question can be asked. The answer will help the organism to overcome the disharmony.

5.3 Herbal extracts

The next chapter describes the most important compresses, poultices and baths. In most of these there is a vegetable matter, usually in the form of a herbal extract (herbal tea) which can also often have a healing effect when taken internally.

The *preparation* of the herbal tea requires some attention. To begin with, it is important to make a distinction between the preparation of different sorts of tea. The purpose of herbal tea is to extract the aromatic and other effective substances from the plant. Depending on the *part* of the plant that is used, the tea requires boiling or brewing for a longer or shorter time. This is necessary so that the required substances are extracted from the plant with as little damage as possible.

Flowers are most closely linked to heat, and need little preparation to release their healing properties. *Leaves* require a little more heat, if the healing substances are to be extracted. *Roots* only release these qualities after lengthy preparation. *Fruit* and *seed* fall between the flower and the root and require comparable preparation.

Thus, increasing amounts of heat and preparation are required for the plants from the flower to the root, in order to extract the substances and qualities from which the human organism can benefit.

THE FOLLOWING RULES APPLY WITH REGARD TO THE PREPARATION OF THE VARIOUS SORTS OF TEA:

FLOWERS (such as camomile) are covered with boiling water and left for one minute. Then sieve.

AROMATIC FRUITS OR SEEDS (such as cumin or aniseed) are placed in boiling water, boiled for half a minute and then left to brew for three to five minutes. Then sieve.

TENDER LEAVES (such as peppermint or birch leaves) are covered with boiling water and left to brew for two to three minutes. Then sieve.

THICK LEAVES (such as barberry or senna leaves). Cover with cold water, bring to the boil and simmer for five minutes. Then leave to brew for five minutes and sieve.

STALKS (for example, equisetum). Cover with cold water, then boil for five to ten minutes and leave to brew for five minutes. Then sieve.

ROOTS AND BARK (for example, calamus and oak bark). Leave to soak in cold water overnight. Bring to the boil and boil gently for five to ten minutes. Then sieve.

HARD SEEDS (such as rosehip). Cover with cold water, boil for five to ten minutes. Leave to brew for five minutes and sieve.

BARLEY WATER. Take 50 g (2 oz) barley grains in 2 litres (2 quarts) of water. Boil for one and a half hours (possibly with a lemon or lemon peel). Add a teaspoonful of honey.

5.4 General remarks

Herbal teas should always be prepared in a saucepan with a lid to prevent the aromatic substances, which are volatile, from evaporating.

When leaving herbal tea to brew keep it warm by using a tea cosy or a tea light.

Always use fresh water, as water from a boiler has been in a metal container for a long time and has lost its vital properties. The herbs should be stored in well sealed jars, in a dark, cool place.

For drinking, use one teaspoonful of herbs per cup and follow the method of preparation described above.

For poultices and compresses, one and a half dessertspoonfuls of the herb per litre (quart) of water is sufficient (unless prescribed otherwise), and three to five minutes should be added to the brewing time described for the preparations above.

For bathing, take a handful of the required herb (unless described otherwise) and leave to brew for five to ten minutes longer than described above.

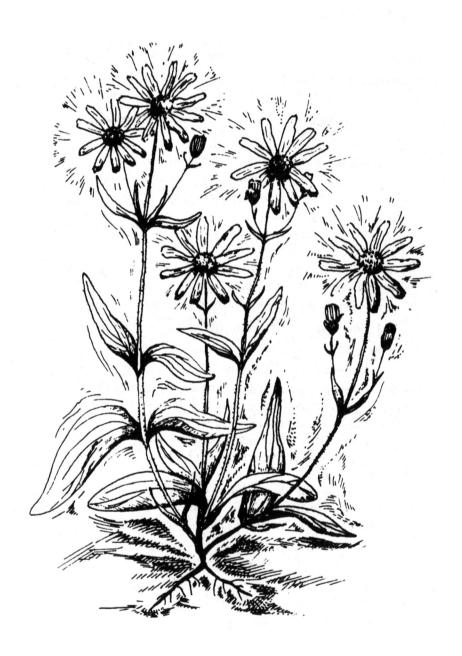

6. Plant Treatments

6.1 *Arnica* (Arnica montana)

The arnica used in medicine comes mainly from the mountains of Central Europe. The plant thrives in wide open spaces with a lot of light and grows best in pebbly soil. It cannot survive in a chalky soil. Artificial fertilizer kills off this plant.

The higher in the mountains the arnica grows, the more aromatic the flower. The leaves grow in pairs of two or three leaves like rosettes, close to the ground. The hairy stalk is almost without leaves, apart from a few much smaller pairs.

Arnica blooms in June or July with a sunny yellowish-orange flower. The 'heart' consists of petals fused together to form a tube, and they radiate in a rather untidy fashion. (It is characteristic of composite flowers to have petals fused into a tube and florets together in one flower.)

When it has flowered, the feathery seeds of this plant are scattered by the autumn wind. The activity above the earth ceases, and activity under the earth begins. The vertical root grows straight, horizontal runners, resulting in a network of roots. The root has a great deal of vitality and continues to survive for a long time, even after the plant above the ground has stopped growing. All the runners on the central root end in a bud from which a new rosette of leaves develops to grow into a new plant the following year. Because of the vitality of the root, one arnica plant produces a number of others.

The plant prefers a cool environment; the pattern of roots reveal the contracting and cold element present in the arnica. When it is applied, this quality comes into its own. It is effective in cases where the fluid processes exceed their limits.

To prepare an extract of arnica or the ointment, the whole plant is used. Externally arnica is used for internal wounds, swellings resulting from bruising, and internal bleeding or bruises.

(a) Compress or fomentation

REQUIREMENTS

- — arnica essence 20 percent
- — unit of measurement, for example, a dessertspoon or a cup
- — bowl
- — compress or fomentation cloth
- — jersey bandage
- — safety pins
- — towel

PROCEDURE

Dilute the 20 percent arnica essence with water in the proportion of one part arnica essence to nine parts water, using a measuring jug. The water may be cool, but should not be ice cold. Soak the compress or bandage in the bowl of liquid.

Now place a towel under the part of the body to be treated. The compress can be taken out of the bowl, pressed out and applied on or around the swollen part. The poultice or compress is held in place with the jersey bandage. To keep the compress damp, a little of the solution can be poured into the bandage with a cup or spoon from time to time.

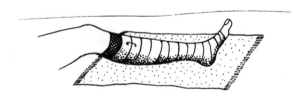

The injured part of the body should rest as much as possible. A sprained or bruised ankle needs to be supported on a chair, or on the sofa. A hand or wrist injury should be supported with a sling. In cases of concussion the fluids collect locally, causing swelling (oedema) of the brain tissue. An arnica compress on the forehead helps soothe the pain and reduce the swelling and bruising.

A patient who is concussed should lie on his back, possibly with one thin pillow; the curtains in the room should be drawn so that the light is dim. Make the arnica solution as described above, place the towel under the patient's head and apply the compress. Make sure that it is not so wet that any drips run down the temples on to the neck.

(b) Treatment with ointment

Arnica (10 percent) ointment is used to treat an injury after the compress or fomentation, as well as for bumps and bruises. The ointment is applied thinly.

(c) Contraindications

Some people may be allergic to arnica. The skin reacts with a localized rash, usually red in colour. In this case, stop the treatment and consult a doctor.

6.2 Stinging nettle (Urtica urens)

The large stinging nettle *(Urtica dioica),* and the small nettle *(Urtica urens)* are both used in medicine. The extract from the small nettle, with an even fiercer sting than the large one, is used for making Combudoron, which is used to treat burns.

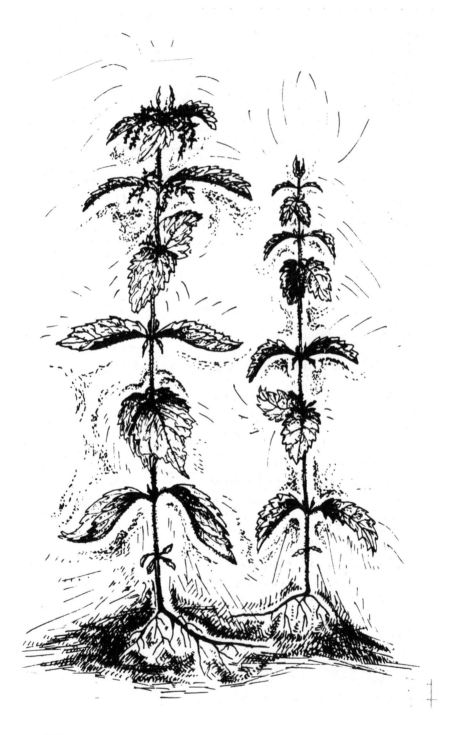

While the large stinging nettle can grow as tall as a man, the small stinging nettle does not grow higher than 50 cm (20 in). Both sorts are very common along roadsides, on rubbish dumps, old walls or open spaces in woods. They prefer a pebbly soil rich in nitrogen. The small nettle prefers a richer soil, near farms, chicken sheds and compost heaps.

The most striking thing about the plant is its leaves. Successive pairs of leaves grow at right angles, the square stem is divided into sections by nodes and these sections are also at right angles to each other. This is a definite pattern.

The leaf of the small stinging nettle has a fairly rounded shape with a short tip. The edges are deeply serrated. The stinging hairs on the leaf release a corrosive fluid when they are touched causing a burning, itchy rash on the skin. Each leaf has two smaller axillary leaves where it joins the stem. At the top of the plant the axillary leaves are replaced by greenish white clusters of flowers, which are not very noticeable and have no smell.

The seed of this plant is very light and can be carried to great heights by the wind. The seeds germinate easily on old, mossy roofs and on ruins.

The straight, yellowish root does not grow runners and the plant is only propagated by seed.

After flowering, in the summer and autumn, the small nettle dies off. The flower of a plant is generally an expression of the element of heat (see Chapter 3). However, the characteristics of the element of heat are lacking in the flower of the stinging nettle. It has no colour, odour or nectar. Its quality of heat can only be felt when the plant is touched. The small nettle encompasses the element of heat within itself.

What is revealed in the plant as a whole, and the way in which it encompasses heat, is also its healing quality when administered, for example, for burns.

A small amount of arnica is added to the medicinal extract, as well as the juice of the whole flowering plant.

(a) Application of the stinging nettle

It is used in ointments for burns and can be used for burns, sunburn, insect bites and itchy skin rashes (hives and shingles).

NOTE: In the case of burns, *immediately* place the affected area under cold, running water for at least five minutes. Watch that the patient does not faint. This is the most important first aid measure to consider in the case of burns. Secondly, a compress can be prepared and applied.

(b) Large or small compress

REQUIREMENTS

— Combudoron lotion
— a measure, such as a dessertspoon or cup
— compress or bandage. This must be ironed to prevent infection
— absorbent surgical bandage
— bowl
— towel

PROCEDURE

Wash your hands thoroughly. Dilute the lotion with cold water in the proportion of one part essence to nine parts water. The cloth is placed in the bowl, the towel under the affected part of the body. Squeeze the moisture out of the compress slightly, and then place on or around the burned skin. Carefully bandage up to keep the compress in position. *On no account* should the

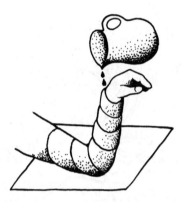

compress be allowed to dry out. Keep it moist by pouring small amounts of the solution between the bandage from time to time: it is not necessary to remove the compress every time as this would increase the chance of infection. The *undiluted* essence can also be patted on hives, chicken-pox and insect bites with some cotton wool. It can also be used undiluted for shingles. As this is a very painful condition, it is better not to pat it on, but to apply it with a spray.

(c) Treatment with ointment

Combudoron ointment or jelly for wounds and burns is used to treat large burns, as well as small, superficial burns, itchy skin rashes and sunburns.

In some cases it is necessary to cover the skin with protective gauze. In this case the ointment or jelly must be applied fairly thickly so that it does not stick to the wound. If this does happen, do *not* tear the gauze off but apply more ointment *over* the piece of gauze that has stuck. The gauze will automatically separate from the skin at a later point.

73

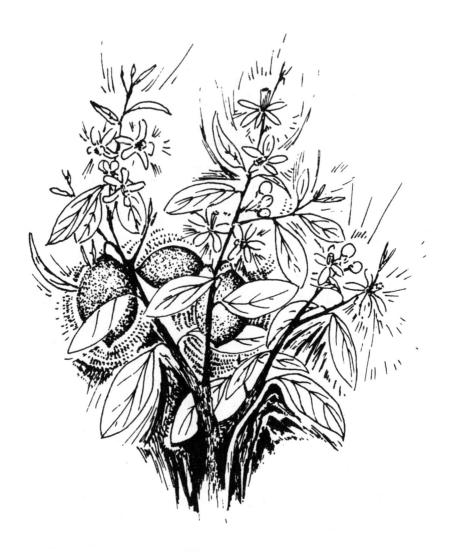

6.3 *Lemons* (Citrus media)

The lemon tree, which grows in the tropics and subtropical areas, is a small, thorny tree with many branches. Just as the tree spreads its branches some distance above the earth, it is

74

also firmly planted in the earth with widely spreading roots. The tree has a large number of dark green leaves, which stay green throughout the year.

When it blossoms, the white flowers spread a sweet and overpowering fragrance. The leaves are also strongly aromatic, though their fragrance is less sweet, less intoxicating and slightly less sharp. The fruit smells fresh and full-bodied, and the thick, rather coarse leathery skin of the lemon is a cool yellow colour. The flesh of the fruit is colourless. On the inside of the skin there is a spongy white pith which has a bitter taste. From the peel to the centre, the lemon is divided into triangular segments by white membranes.

Despite the hot climate, the flesh of the fruit does not produce fructose, as one might expect, but remains sour. The seeds (pips) of the lemon are surrounded by a bitter, slimy substance.

When we examine the plant in its totality, it is noticeable that the outward turned character of the flowers is reversed in the fruit and metamorphosed into a strictly ordered, contracting principle. In medicine, the lemon repeats this process in conditions in which excessive metabolic activity has arisen in an area where this should not occur, that is, wherever excessive heat processes need to be limited and restrained.

(a) Use of lemons

Compresses with lemon juice on the feet and lower parts of the leg are often given when a patient is in danger of losing consciousness as a result of fever, or starts to become delirious. The excessive heat of the head must be conducted to the legs. The following treatment can be very effective.

(b) Compress for the legs

Use only if the feet are very hot.

— a bowl of lukewarm water
— one lemon
— a knife
— a cloth
— for small children, a few pairs of large socks
— 2 towels
— 2 safety pins

PROCEDURE

The lemon is cut in half and one half is placed in the bowl of lukewarm water. It is cut into a star shape under water and then the juice is pressed out. In this way both the juice and the volatile etheric oil from the skin is released into the water.

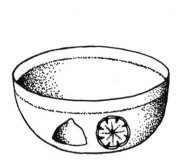 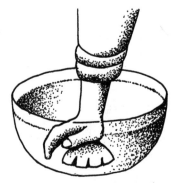

The cloth for the compress is rolled up and placed in the bowl.

The blankets are turned back at the foot of the bed and folded back. One towel is placed under each leg. The legs should be bare

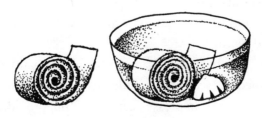

to just above the knees. One roll is now thoroughly squeezed so that not a drop remains in the compress, and then it is wound round the leg from the toe to the knee. Make sure that there are no gaps and that the whole foot is thoroughly wrapped up. The towel under the leg is folded and pinned around the foot and the leg. A woollen shawl can also be used as a bandage around the compress. For small children it is usually easier to fit a large cotton or woollen sock over the compress.

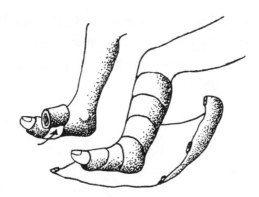

The other foot and leg are then wrapped up in the same way and the bedclothes are replaced.

After twenty to twenty-five minutes the compresses will have dried out. If they have not, they were probably too wet when they were applied, and the patient may even have got cold feet. In this case, the compresses should be removed immediately and the feet can be warmed with a hot water bottle or rubbed warm.

Depending on the patient's condition, the treatment can be repeated immediately or after a little while. If he has fallen into a peaceful sleep, the compresses can be left on, provided you are sure that they have dried out. If the process is repeated, use the other half of the lemon and fresh water.

(c) Chest compress (for bronchitis)

REQUIREMENTS

— a bowl
— boiling water
— knife and fork
— one lemon
— woollen material, which goes round the chest easily
— a bandage, which goes round the chest easily
— another piece of material, which goes round the chest easily
— a cloth to wring out
— safety pins

PROCEDURE

The room temperature should be comfortable and the windows kept shut. The patient should go to the toilet before the treatment. The bed is prepared as follows: the woollen material with the safety pins attached is placed behind the patient's back. Another piece of material is placed on the woollen material. The bandage is folded to size and rolled to the centre from two sides. This is placed on the cloth to wring out, and this too is rolled up, so that there are two 'ears' at each end of it.

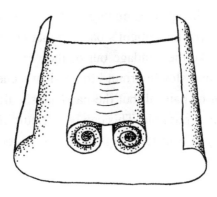

The patient bares his chest and is then tucked up, taking care the shoulders are also under the covers.

For this treatment use a whole lemon. The boiling water is poured into the bowl, and using a knife and fork, cut the two halves into star shapes under water. Then the two halves are pressed out, for instance with the base of a cup. The cloths are placed in the bowl, holding on to the ears so that these remain dry. Leave the boiling water with lemon juice to soak into the cloths thoroughly. Then wring them out quickly and firmly, still holding onto the ears. No drips should come out of the cloth when you have finished.

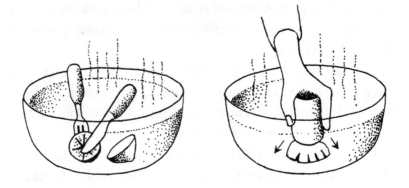

The patient now sits up for a minute. Leaving the bandage in the wrung-out cloth, pat the patient's back so that he can get used to the heat. Then take the bandage out of the wrung out cloth and roll it carefully and slowly around the patient's chest. The treatment should not be painful, but the bandage should nevertheless be applied as hot as possible. This can be difficult, especially with children, but if you wait too long, the bandage cools down very quickly.

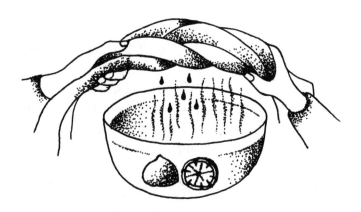

When the bandage has been rolled round the chest, another cloth and the woollen cloth are tied round and fastened with a safety pin. The patient then puts on a cardigan or pyjama top and is thoroughly tucked in.

The compress should remain fastened for at least twenty to thirty minutes, unless the patient feels uncomfortable, or it has gone cold. Then it should be removed earlier. If the cloth was too moist it will cool down very quickly.

If the patient falls asleep, this means that the treatment was effective and the compress can be left. Otherwise, the cloths should be removed quickly and the patient given warm clothes to wear. Because of the big differences in temperature, it is absolutely essential that everything is laid out ready to wear before the clothes are removed, so that the patient does not become cold. After the treatment, the patient should rest for a while.

(d) Compress for the throat

Use for a sore throat.

REQUIREMENTS

As described above, but this time to fit around the neck.

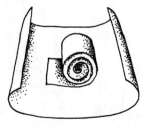

PROCEDURE

As described above. The compress is rolled in one direction only.

(e) Colds

Colds, in which the mucous membrane of the nose and throat is irritated, can be treated by putting a slice of lemon under the soles of the feet, and keeping this in place with a sock or small bandage. This can be left in place all night and the treatment can be repeated the following night if necessary. This simple treatment leads the excessive metabolic activity of the nose and throat to the lower regions, and the properties of the lemon act as an example of this.

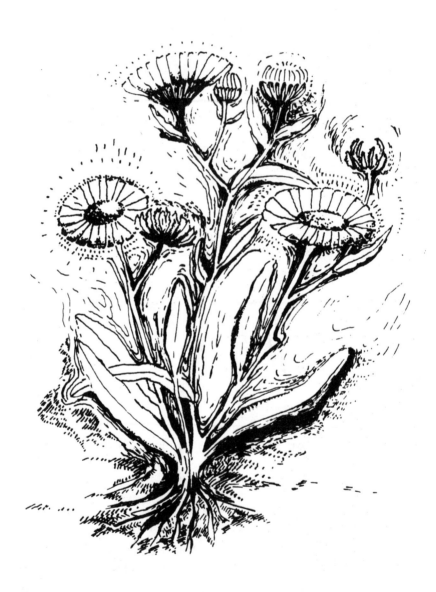

6.4 The marigold (Calendula officinalis)

The marigold originates from the Mediterranean countries, where it flowers throughout the year. Since the Middle Ages the marigold has been a common domestic flower in more northern regions as well, where it flowers from June to late autumn.

The plant seeds itself and soon takes over. The seed germinates easily. Within a short while it grows into a plant with many, fairly fleshy, elongated leaves. The leaves contain a great deal of moisture and the lower leaves are often spongy.

Vivid, orange flowers appear from the thick round buds. The heart of the flower consists of petals fused to form a tube, and the petals radiate from this in a strict pattern. Although the plant flowers for a long time, each individual flower only lasts a few days. The flowers open at sunrise so that they follow the movement of the sun and thus absorb the rays; in the evening the petals close up again. When they are to be used for medicinal purposes, the flowers should be picked early in the morning before they open up.

A striking feature of this plant is the contrast between the riotous, rather untidy leaves, and the strictly developed flower. In the flower, the plant conquers the chaotic disorderly character, typical of the leaves. This can be considered as symbolizing the effect of calendula as a medicinal plant.

(a) The use of calendula

Calendula can stimulate 'dirty wounds' to heal, so that new tissue can be formed. In the end the wound can be assimilated into the rest of the organism.

(b) Large or small compress

REQUIREMENTS

- calendula lotion (20 percent)
- a measuring jug
- a bowl
- a compress or a piece of cloth
- an absorbent bandage or gauze to hold the compress in place
- a towel

PROCEDURE

Wash the hands thoroughly. Dilute one part calendula lotion with nine parts tepid water, using a measuring jug. Place the compress or cloth in the bowl. Place a towel under the part of the body to be treated, to protect the bedding. The cloth is then wrung out slightly and placed on the wound, still very damp. Finally, put on the bandage to keep the compress in place. The compress should not dry out, so a small amount of calendula lotion should be poured regularly on to the bandage. The cloth

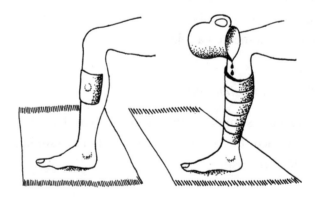

itself should be replaced regularly because of the infected wound.

Throw away old cloths after using them, and disinfect any materials still to be used with a disinfectant, and then boil them.

When the wound is clean and new tissue has formed, which can be seen from the small pink border round the edge of the wound, you can continue by using calendula ointment, as continuous wet compresses could soften the new tissue.

(c) Treatment with ointment

Wash your hands thoroughly and put some calendula ointment or jelly on a piece of gauze or plaster, if necessary with an applicator. This treatment can be used for minor grazes, infected cuticles and nappy rash in babies.

6.5 *Camomile* (Matricaria chamomilla)

Matricaria chamomilla grows by the roadside, on building sites and amidst rubble. It does not require a soil rich in humus, but poor, chalky soil. It also needs light, air and sun. Camomile cannot survive in shade or a damp environment.

The seeds fall out in autumn and develop into a leaf rosette with finely feathered flowers. It remains dormant through the winter and in the first warmth of spring the rosette grows into a full, bushy plant with double feathered leaves, with the bases fairly far apart. The sun can shine right down to the foot of the plant through this fine network of leaves.

A cross-section of the leaves reveals that the borders are rolled down, which means that the leaf, though it appears very light, still contains a lot of mesophyll.

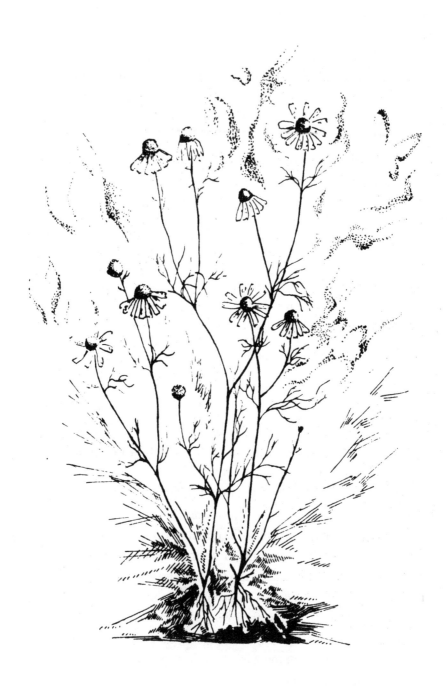

The long-stemmed flower-heads consist of petals fused together to form a tube. The tall, warm yellow heart is hollow inside. In this it is distinct from other types of camomile. The white florets turn down when they have been in the sun for a while, so that the high, cone-shaped heart is even more striking. Camomile flowers profusely from the spring to the autumn. The volatile, etheric oil from the flowers has a blue colour, not yellow or reddish yellow like most etheric oils.

The camomile plant is totally saturated with light, air and sun. It assimilates the warmth completely and is able to do so because it has control over warmth. Hence camomile has a relaxing and regulating effect in complaints in which the healing mechanism is disturbed.

(a) Uses of camomile

Camomile has a calming effect. It is used for many conditions, including nausea, stomach upset and period pains.

(b) Compress for the stomach

REQUIREMENTS

— a piece of woollen material
— safety pins
— a cloth for the compress
— another piece of cloth
— a cloth to wring out
— a saucepan and lid
— a large sieve
— camomile flowers
— a large bowl or deep dish
— a hot water bottle

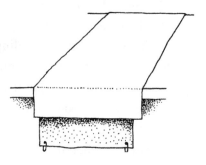

PROCEDURE

The patient should go to the toilet or be helped to go (see Sections 4.2 (a) and (b)). The room should be at a comfortable temperature and the windows should be shut. The bedside table is cleared. The bed is prepared by placing the piece of woollen material with the safety pins attached, about halfway down the under-sheet and placing another piece of cloth on top of this.

The patient lies down in bed and has one or two pillows under his head. Make sure the cloths are in the right place and are the right size. The compress cloth is rolled in from two ends and

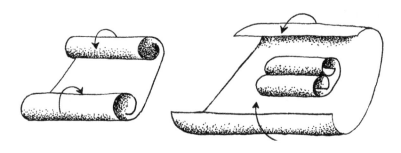

rolled up in the wringing out cloth so that two 'ears' remain on the sides of the wringing out cloth, which can be held later when the compress is wrung out. Place this in the bowl.

The patient's top clothes are pulled up a little; the lower clothes are pulled down. He is then warmly tucked in, and if he has cold feet, he is given a hot water bottle.

The tea is made by boiling about a litre (quart) of cold water. A small handful of camomile flowers is added and the pan is taken off the heat so that the tea can brew for about two minutes. The tea is then poured through the sieve into the bowl, in which the rolled up cloth has already been placed. Make sure the 'ears' remain dry, when the inner cloth is thoroughly soaked.

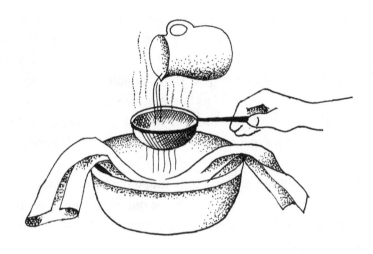

The cloths are then wrung out quickly and firmly to the extent that no further moisture can be wrung out. This is important as a compress, which is too wet, cools down very quickly and apart from the effect of the cold, it feels extremely uncomfortable. The patient sits up and the rolled up cloth is patted against his back so that the skin can get used to the heat.

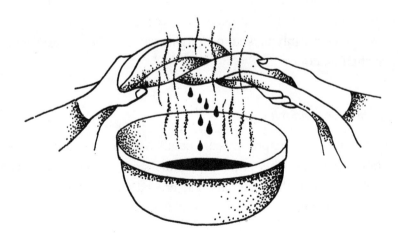

The wringing cloth is then removed, the compress is again patted against the patient's back and placed behind the patient and rolled out a little way. The patient lies down on it carefully and first one side is rolled over the stomach and then the other. The compress should be applied as hot as possible without hurting the patient. Finally, the extra cloth and the piece of woollen material are folded over the patient and the whole thing is fastened with safety pins.

The cloths should be tied firmly round the body. If they are too loose the compress will cool down too quickly. A hot water bottle with just a little water, placed on the stomach, helps to keep the compress warm.

Cover the patient up warmly, making sure that the shoulders and feet are also tucked in. At the risk of stating the obvious, it should be stressed that this treatment, which is based on heat, should always be very hot. So the treatment must be properly prepared and administered quickly.

The compress stays in place for twenty to thirty minutes. If the patient falls asleep, the cloths can stay where they are, because if they have been effective, they will dry out by themselves.

If the cloths are removed after a while, the large difference in temperature should be taken into account. The patient must therefore be warmly tucked in straightaway and should rest for at least half an hour.

(c) Smaller stomach compress

For this type of compress, use a smaller cloth, folded double a number of times. This is placed on the stomach (not round it). Apart from this, the materials and procedures are the same as described above.

CONTRAINDICATIONS

If you have any doubts regarding the nature of the stomach-ache
it is better not to give this treatment, but to consult a doctor. For
diarrhoea or a stomach-ache with a fever, the hot fomentation or
compress should not be given either, unless the doctor advises
this.

(d) Inhalation

A cold, which will not move, can be treated with a inhalation of
camomile tea. The vapour of the camomile affects the mucous
membrane of the nose and throat when it is breathed in, and helps
to stimulate the slowed down metabolic processes in the upper
half of the body.

REQUIREMENTS

- a large towel or sheet
- another towel or scarf
- a large bowl
- camomile flowers
- boiling water

PROCEDURE

The room where the inhalation is to be taken should be comfortably warm with windows and doors shut. It is best if the patient
sits at a table next to the bed. His hair should be covered with
a towel or scarf, and then a large bath towel, or a sheet folded
double, is placed over his head and shoulders. Make sure his
feet are warm; he should be wearing socks or slippers, or the
feet could be placed on a hot water bottle, and a rug laid round
the legs and feet.

Scatter a handful of camomile flowers in the bowl and pour about a litre (quart) of boiling water over these. The bowl is immediately placed on the table in front of the patient and the towel or sheet is laid over the bowl so that it is completely encased, and no air can enter from outside. The patient breathes in the vapours. The inhalation lasts ten to twenty minutes. Then remove the bowl, dry the patient's face and put him back to bed. A clean towel should be placed round his head to prevent him cooling down too quickly. Make sure the patient has handkerchiefs and give him a bag where he can put the used ones.

If this treatment has been carried out properly, the patient will feel as though there is air and space inside his head once again. However, the danger of an inhalation is that the patient could catch another cold as a result of the change in temperature.

PREVENTION OF COLDS

Many people are susceptible to the cold, especially as regards their air passages. One important cause of this is that the air in centrally-heated houses is often much too dry, so that the mucous membrane, especially of the air passages, dries out. This increases their sensitivity.

As a preventative measure, place a bowl of water containing a few drops of eucalyptus oil on the bedroom radiators. As the water warms up, the oil slowly evaporates so that there is an even humidity level throughout the air.

(e) Enema

An enema with camomile tea can be given for various reasons, as a laxative or to cure the irritated lining of the intestines. However, it is advisable only to give this sort of treatment after consulting the doctor, or if it has been prescribed. A few practical guidelines are given below for these cases.

REQUIREMENTS

   — a piece of rubber or plastic to protect the lower sheet
   — a towel
   — an irrigator, syringe or balloon
   — a large bowl
   — a sieve
   — a saucepan and lid
   — bath thermometer
   — vaseline

PROCEDURE

Bring half a litre of water to the boil and add a handful of camomile flowers. Remove the pan from the heat straightaway, cover with the lid and leave to brew for one or two minutes. Then sieve. The tea is now left to cool to body temperature (37°C, 98.6°F). You can continue with the other preparations for the treatment. The patient should go to the toilet or be given the bedpan (see Sections 4.2 (a) and (b)). Place the rubber or plastic sheeting behind, and partially under, the patient's buttocks, and cover with a towel. The rubber or plastic serves to protect the lower sheet; the towel is used because the patient feels cold.

Whatever instrument is used to introduce the tea into the intestines, it is important to check that the syringe is not too stiff, the rubber is still all right, and so on. The end, which is placed in the anus, is first coated with vaseline. Use the thermometer to measure the temperature of the camomile tea. It should be exactly

37°C (98.6°F). Fill the instrument and fix the cannula to the end. The patient lies on his left side with his legs slightly drawn up. Then put the cannula into the anus and slide it 5 to 10 cm (2 to 4 in) inside (5 cm for children; 10 cm for adults), but certainly no further.

Ask the patient to take a few deep sighs when it is introduced, as this relaxes him and simplifies the treatment.

The tea should be introduced *slowly.* If a syringe is used, press the plunger slowly. A balloon is pressed slowly and gradually, and if an irrigator is used, this should not be placed too high above the patient.

When all the tea has entered the intestines, press the cannula tightly shut and remove from the anus. Leave the rubber sheeting and the towel, but clear away the rest of the materials used. Clean with hot soda water and if necessary, with a disinfectant.

It is best if the patient can retain the tea as long as possible — at least for ten minutes. Then give him the bedpan or help him go to the toilet. It is essential to stay with the patient. He may feel unwell with intestinal cramps.

(f) Inhalation for a chill on the bladder

When the patient has a chill on the bladder, this leads to frequent urination in which only small amounts of urine are released, and it becomes painful. This can be treated with a camomile inhalation.

REQUIREMENTS

- a blanket or thick flannel sheet
- camomile flowers
- a dish or pan
- boiling water

PROCEDURE

Place a handful of camomile flowers in the dish or pan. These are covered with boiling water and then placed or hung inside the toilet bowl. The patient then sits down on the toilet with the blanket or flannel right over him so that he is covered up from head to toe. Keep the feet warm with slippers, woollen socks or a hot water bottle. Remain seated for ten minutes and then quickly put on a pair of pyjama trousers and go to bed. This treatment can be repeated on two or three evenings.

If the pain has still not disappeared, consult the doctor.

(g) Toothache

A rinse with camomile tea has a soothing effect on toothache. It is also possible to place a small compress on the aching tooth. Use a piece of gauze or a thin piece of cloth. Place the compress in a sieve and hold over the steam of boiling water for a moment so that the flowers are moist. Then place the compress under the aching tooth between the gum and the cheek.

Ready-to-use camomile tea bags are convenient and easy to use for this purpose. When they have been held over the steam for a moment they can be placed on the painful spot.

6.6 *Horseradish* (Cochlearia armoracia)

Usually, this large plant is cultivated for its root, but it also grows wild. It does best in a sandy, moist soil. In the fully grown plant two sorts of leaves can be distinguished as regards their position: the root leaves, which grow directly from the root, and the leaves which grow on the stalk. The root leaves, which can grow up to a metre long, are coarsely and irregularly serrated. It is only when the root of the plant is fully grown that the horseradish develops

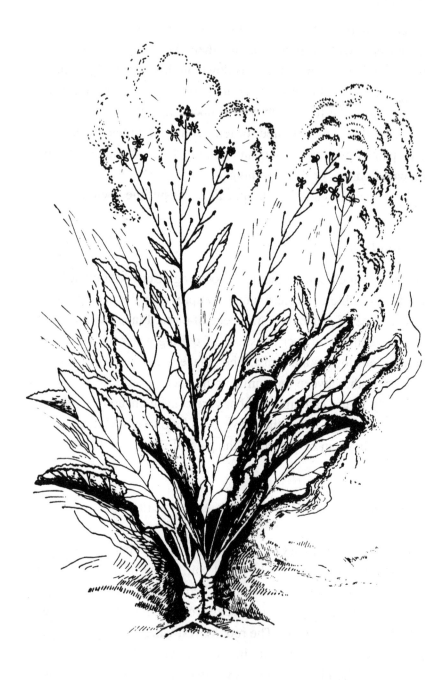

a flowering stalk in the spring and the stalk leaves grow on this. These are much smaller than the root leaves and are slightly feathery. In the autumn the plant loses all its leaves.

At the end of the flowering stalk, the horseradish plant has a clump of small, strongly-scented white flowers. The seed of these flowers seldom ripens.

The strength of the plant is particularly centred in the root, with which it propagates itself by means of runners. The root has a sharp, spicy taste, reminiscent of pepper, and the plant is rich in vitamin C. The whole plant — but especially the root — contains etheric oil, a so-called mustard oil, which is sharp, biting and peppery. The root, the coolest part of the plant (see Chapter 3), actually has a characteristic hot quality in the horseradish plant. If it were compared to a person, it could be said that the metabolic processes are taking place in the nervous/sensory area. The oil from the root leads to increased circulation in the skin (nervous/sensory area) as well as heat (hyperaemia), and removes trapped metabolic processes from their isolation.

(a) The uses of the horseradish plant

Inflammation, which occurs in cavities in the body, the nasal and frontal sinuses, can be diffused by being treated externally with horseradish. By applying the sharp oil, which is formed in this root, to the skin, a sort of external inflammation is provoked so that the internal inflammatory processes are led outwards.

This makes it possible to recover the balance between the inflammatory and hardening processes in the upper and lower regions of the body respectively. In other words, by using the horseradish plant to free the excess of metabolic processes 'trapped' in the wrong place, the rhythmic system can keep the balance of the opposite processes there.

(b) Compress for sinusitis

R<small>EQUIREMENTS</small>

- — fresh horseradish
- — a flat grater
- — a saucer
- — a small knife
- — a cloth for the compress
- — vaseline
- — a plaster

P<small>ROCEDURE</small>

In general the patient can adopt the position he finds most comfortable. Draughts and cold should certainly be avoided, and warm feet are important.

Take a small piece of the root, rinse clean if necessary, and scrape off a little of the peel. Then grate some of the root over a saucer. To treat a case of sinusitis, you need about half a teaspoonful of grated root. This is placed in the middle of the compress, and then all the edges are folded over and stuck down with a plaster.

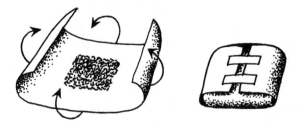

The compress is put in place and held there by the patient himself. For the treatment of sinusitis, some vaseline is applied to two small pieces of cloth or gauze, and these are then 'stuck' down over the patient's eyes to prevent them watering too much, and to avoid irritation from the sharp odour.

After a while, depending on the freshness of the root and the sensitivity of the skin, the patient will become aware of a burning feeling. The compress can be removed for a moment and then replaced until the effect of the root diminishes. Then the cloths can be rinsed out, and if necessary, used again.

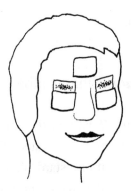

The treatment with horseradish should not be given more than once a day, at most. Always begin with a short treatment to find out how fresh the root is and how the skin of the patient reacts. Sometimes the sharp heat continues to have an effect for a long time, and can even result in burns.

Because of the danger of burns it is advisable for the patient to hold the compress himself. Depending on how he feels, he can remove it immediately. The compress should *never* be stuck down.

Fresh horseradish is only available in the autumn and winter. It can be kept in a flowerpot filled with earth, or be wrapped up in a paper bag and stored in the vegetable compartment of the fridge.

If there is no fresh horseradish available, it is also possible to use powdered horseradish. However, this is not as strong, but the danger of burns is considerably reduced. (Patients who react violently to fresh horseradish can therefore be treated with powdered horseradish as an alternative.)

To use the powder, put two teaspoonfuls with a little water in a glass or cup, and stir until there is an even consistency. This is sufficient for one compress when it has been applied to the cloth and taped up with a plaster.

Compresses made with powder are usually tolerated for a longer time on the skin.

6.7 *The mustard plant* (Sinapis alba *and* Sinapis nigra)

The white mustard plant *(Sinapis alba)* and the black mustard plant *(Sinapis nigra)* are both cultivated, though they are also found in the wild. The white mustard plant is rather rare in the wild, but the black mustard plant is quite common, and grows particularly well in poor, salty soil.

The plant needs an open and light environment. Light is a more important factor than heat for the survival of this plant and, therefore, it is found in the far north but does not grow in the tropics.

The black mustard plant is a large, striking plant, which can grow 80 to 100 cm (30 to 40 in) tall. The white mustard plant is slightly smaller.

The leaves are large and irregularly serrated, but the upper leaves are small and narrow.

Both varieties have rather sweet-smelling, yellow flowers, which are very popular with bees. The mustard plants owe their name to the colour of the seed; the white mustard plant produces creamy seeds; the black mustard plant produces

100

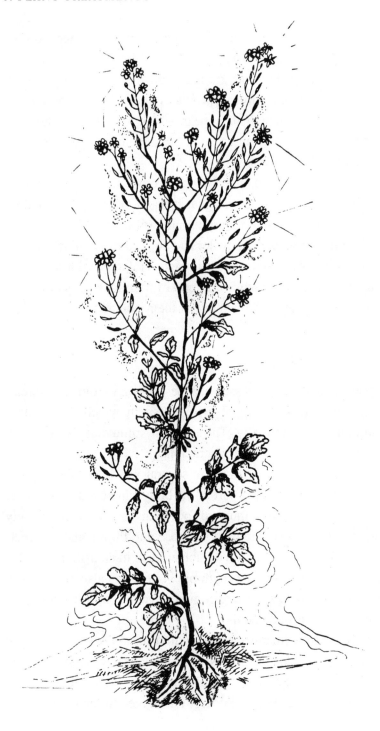

small, brownish-black seeds. The seed is rich in etheric oil, or mustard oil, which is sharp, piquant and fiery.

The mustard plant grows from a small seed to a strong plant in a fairly short space of time. It produces buds, flowers and goes to seed. Meanwhile, new buds appear, which also flower. Thus, the plant has buds, flowers and seed at the same time. This is characteristic of many flowers.

The fact that the plant can go through these processes so quickly in a poor soil reveals that it has a great deal of vitality, which is expressed in the sharp burning oil of the seed.

When it is ground to a powder and applied to the skin, the seed has a strong effect and the skin reacts violently with a flow of blood and heat (hyperaemia). Internal inflammations can be dissipated in this way and taken out of their isolation.

(a) The uses of mustard

Trapped metabolic processes can be removed from the 'threatened' area with the help of a treatment in which the mustard is administered externally. The mustard stimulates the skin and leads to better circulation (hyperaemia).

This process can take place in several ways. Metabolic processes trapped in the upper part of the body can be led to the lower areas with the help of a mustard foot-bath (migraine, chronically swollen mucous membrane of the nose and throat, and the treatment can be supplemental with horseradish in sinusitis). Trapped metabolic processes in the rhythmic system can also be led away from the trunk with a mustard compress on the chest (for instance, for bronchitis or pneumonia).

As treatment with mustard does entail certain risks, it should be stressed that the doctor must be consulted, or have recommended the treatment. A few practical guidelines are given below to minimize risks in cases where a doctor has agreed to the treatment.

(b) Chest compress

REQUIREMENTS

— Three handfuls of ground mustard seed. This should all be used. If black ground mustard seed is used, use half this amount. In either case, use half of these amounts for treating children.
— a large cotton compress cloth, which easily goes round the chest
— 2 safety pins
— a large bowl
— 1 ordinary towel
— 2 cloths for the armpits
— 2 cloths for the nipples (also for men)
— vaseline
— an alarm clock or watch

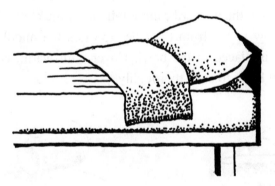

PROCEDURE

The room where the treatment is given should be comfortably warm and the windows should be shut. The patient should go to the toilet or be given the bedpan (see Section 4.2 (a) and (b)) before the treatment. Clear the bedside table.

The bed is made as follows: 1 pillow covered with a towel and the 2 cloths for the armpits are laid on the bedside table, and

103

some vaseline is applied to the cloths for the nipples (for men and women). The large bath towel is placed behind the patient's back with the safety pins attached. Make sure that the cloths fit easily around the patient's chest.

The large compress cloth is laid on a table and the amount of mustard indicated above is placed on it. This is spread out with

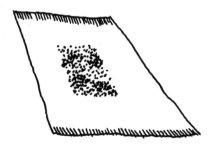

the hands so that there is an even layer in the middle of the cloth. The top, bottom and sides are folded over, covering each other amply, so that the mustard cannot fall out of the cloth. The whole thing is now rolled from the sides towards the middle and this thick roll is placed in the bowl. Cover with warm, not too hot water, and leave to soak thoroughly.

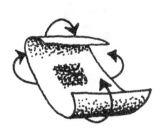 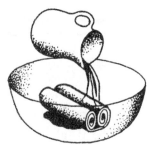

Then wring out the roll carefully, until no more moisture can be squeezed out. (Be careful, as the cloth can easily tear.) The water, which is now yellow, is thrown away, and the roll is placed back in the bowl and taken to the patient.

The patient sits up and bares his chest. The roll is placed behind his back in such a way that there will be one layer of material between the skin and the mustard. It is then rolled out

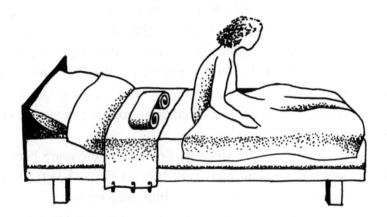

a little, the patient lies down on it, two cloths are placed in his armpits, the two pads are placed on the nipples with vaseline and the compress is wrapped round the chest.

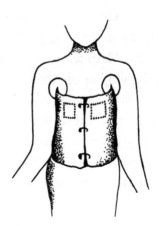

Finally, fold the bath towel round the patient and secure it with safety pins. Tuck the patient's shoulders up with the towel lying on the pillow and then cover him with the rest of the bedclothes.

Make a note of the time and stay in the room. This is very important because if the patient starts to feel a burning sensation, the compress should be removed immediately. This will happen within a few minutes if black mustard powder is used. White mustard powder sometimes takes a little longer, depending on how fresh it is. To prevent burns, the first time this treatment is given, it is advisable to remove the compress after a few minutes, regardless of whether or not the patient feels a burning sensation.

Every skin reacts individually. Sometimes there are burns, even though the patient feels very little at first. The effect of mustard can continue for a long time, and sometimes burns can even appear a few hours later. It is therefore essential to be careful.

Remove the compress quickly, taking care that the patient does not become cold. When you have some practice and can do it quickly, pass a damp face flannel lightly over the treated skin a few times. Then quickly rub some oil lightly into the skin, for instance carob oil, and help the patient to dress; tuck him up warmly, especially the shoulders. Make sure he gets plenty of rest. If there are burns, despite the precautions, it is best to treat the skin with special jelly or ointment for burns.

NOTE: Mustard powder should be stored in well-sealed jars. if you wish to grind the mustard seed yourself, it is best to do this by hand. An electric grinder can catch fire when the etheric oil is released from the seed.

Compresses should be thoroughly rinsed. Then empty the bucket into the toilet.

(c) Small compress

For a small compress, press a proportionate amount of mustard powder on a smaller cloth, and put it where the doctor has indicated. Apart from this, the materials and procedure are the same as described above.

(d) Foot-bath

In the case of migraine the metabolic processes have spread to the upper regions of the body to an extreme extent. The headache, which can even be accompanied by nausea, can be cured with the help of mustard foot-baths. In this way the metabolic processes are led down to the lower half of the body.

REQUIREMENTS

— mustard powder. For adults, use two or three handfuls of white mustard powder or one or two handfuls of black mustard powder. For children, use half of these amounts in both cases.
— a foot-bath
— a towel
— a bath thermometer

PROCEDURE

The foot-bath that is used should be large enough for the patient's feet to fit inside it in a normal position, and should be tall enough for the edge of the bath to go up to the knees. Though it is normally known as a foot-bath, it would be more accurate to call it a lower-leg bath. If necessary, use two buckets and place one leg in each bucket.

The foot-bath or buckets should be placed, if possible, in the bathtub or shower, or otherwise on a mat or floor-cloth. Fill the foot-bath two-thirds full with water and check with a bath thermometer that the temperature is 37°C (98.6°F). Now add the mustard powder and stir into the water until no lumps remain. The patient sits down on a chair or on the edge of the bath and puts his feet in the bath. Make sure that rolled-up trouser legs are not constricting. Cover the patient's shoulders, support his back, and place the towel over his knees so that it also falls over the edge of the foot-bath. This helps the knees to keep warm or to warm up, prevents the water from cooling down too quickly, and means that the patient will not breathe in mustard vapour, which could make him feel sick.

The temperature of the water must not fall below 37°C (98.6°F), so add a little hot water to the foot-bath from time to time.

This treatment lasts fifteen to twenty minutes, though it obviously depends on the patient's condition, the strength of the mustard powder, and therefore the effect on the skin. Mustard foot-baths can also result in burns if too much mustard is used, or if the temperature of the water is too hot. Make sure that the foot-bath does not last any longer than the patient can stand. After the treatment, rinse the remains of the mustard off the leg with warm water; be sure to rinse thoroughly and dry between the toes. Then it is best for the patient to put on some socks and have a rest in bed, if necessary, with a hot water bottle. Draw the curtains and shut out as much noise as possible so that the senses can also come to rest. The foot-bath should be emptied into the toilet.

6.8 Onion (Allium cepa)

The onion originates from the East, though this plant has been grown throughout the world for centuries as a source of food. The bulb of the onion consists of similarly-shaped layers, each of which is covered with a transparent, silky membrane. The outer skin is papery and impermeable.

The onion's roots are small and do not grow deeply into the earth. The onion does not flower in its first year. A few tubular leaves form in the spring, just above the earth. The onion concentrates all its strength in the bulb, and the flowering stalk, which has no leaves, does not shoot up until the second year. The spherical, greenish-white flower blooms at the end of this stalk, consisting of many small star-shaped florets. The whole plant is permeated with a strong characteristic garlicky smell. The whole plant, especially the bulb, has a high content of sulphur, which stimulates the metabolic processes in man.

One might expect an extravagant and colourful flower in a plant which has this quality of stimulating the metabolic processes (see Chapter 3), but this is not the case with Allium cepa. The strength of the onion is revealed in the layers of the bulb, and especially in its powerfully-formed flower. With this strength it is able to control the abundance of sulphur. The strength of form of the onion can be used to overcome the process of inflammation, especially for inflammations in the head and chest area, which correspond to the area where the bulb of the onion grows between the roots and the leaves, the area which is most strongly developed in this plant.

(a) Use of the onion

The above description of the onion's qualities shows that if onion is applied externally, it can be used to break down an inflammation process. The onion acts as an example for the

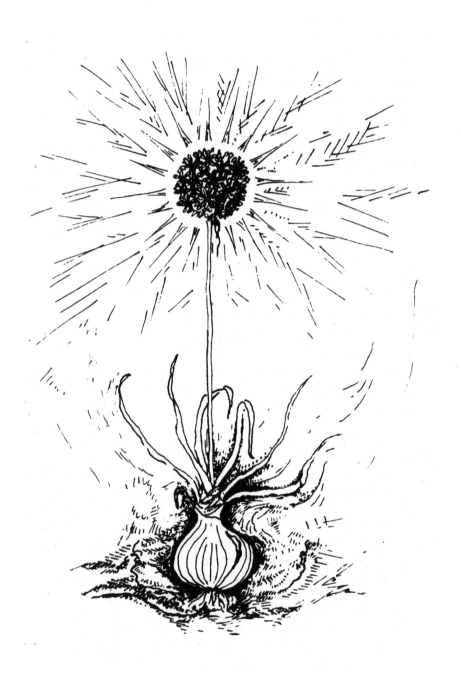

organism of how to deal with the qualities of sulphur and form. An onion compress can be used, for example, in cases of ear infections or inflammation of the joints.

(b) Compress

REQUIREMENTS

- — an onion
- — a knife
- — a chopping board
- — a cloth for the compress
- — a plaster
- — a bandage
- — for earache, normal saline solution (0.9 percent) and a pipette

PROCEDURE

Cut the onion into small pieces, place in the middle of the compress and fold over the edges; stick down at the back with a piece of plaster so that no pieces of onion can fall out of the compress. The compress is placed in the correct position, on or behind the ear, and kept in place with a bandage.

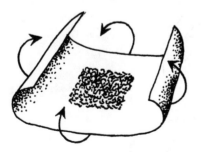
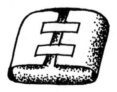

This is often a problem with children. In this case you can simply hold it in place, using a nappy (diaper) as a scarf, crossing over under the chin and securing round the back of the neck.

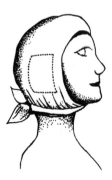

Leave the compress in place for a few hours. The compress or bandage should never be stuck down on the skin with plasters where there is any inflammation, whether internal or external, as this could lead to irritation of the skin.

NOTE: In the case of earache use nose-drops of normal saline solution at least four times a day to keep the eustachian tube free; in this way the accumulated inflamed matter can drain away from the middle ear. (This solution is available from chemists.)

For an inflammation of a joint or ligament it is possible to use a large onion, bruise the layers slightly and place them on

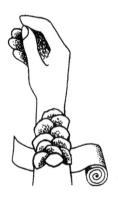

the skin overlapping one another. In this case there is no need to use a cloth, only a bandage to keep them in place.

In general, an onion compress will quickly reduce the pain. If it does not do so, consult the doctor. Particularly with earache, do not wait too long as this may cause serious damage to the inner ear.

7. Other External Treatments

7.1 Curd cheese (quark)

Curd cheese, or quark, is made by leaving fresh milk to go off. After a while the milk separates into a thick, sour mass (the curds) and a yellowish, neutral substance (the whey). The curds and the whey reflect the upper (nervous) and lower (metabolic) poles of the human being. In the treatment, the curd cheese dries out, producing a 'suction effect,' which creates a space where an equilibrium can develop.

With an inflammation (bronchitis, boils, mastitis) the metabolic processes intrude outside their region. The curd cheese treatment allows the processes of the upper pole to have a healing effect (through the curds), so that a balance develops between them. On the other hand, with a dry cough (asthma) the opposite has happened: the forming tendency of the upper (nervous/sensory) pole is 'stuck' in the rhythmic system, leading to a condition of cramp. Again curd cheese can help, this time the whey creating space for the metabolic processes to work.

(a) Chest compress

REQUIREMENTS

- — curd cheese (children 250 g, 8 oz; adults 500 g, 1 lb)
- — a scraper or spoon
- — two hot water bottles
- — a large cotton cloth, which easily fits round the chest (when folded)

— a large towel folded double, which easily fits round
  the chest
— another towel
— two safety pins
— a piece of rubber sheeting or plastic
— a thick flannel sheet

PROCEDURE

To warm up the curd cheese, place the sealed container between
two hot water bottles, or in a pan of hot water. Heating takes at
least ten to fifteen minutes. Meanwhile, everything is prepared
for the treatment, so the windows are shut and the room should
be perfectly warm. Protect the bed with rubber sheeting and
some thick flannel. Make sure that the compress cloth and the
towel are the correct size. The patient should go to the toilet
before the treatment.

When the curd cheese is at body temperature, the container
is taken out of the pan, or removed from between the hot water
bottles. The cloth is placed on the hot water bottles and the curd
cheese is applied to the cloth.

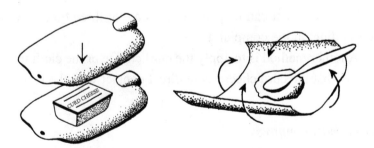

When the curd cheese has been spread evenly over the cloth,
fold over the top, bottom and both sides. The cloth should still fit
around the patient's chest after folding. The whole thing can be

carefully rolled up, put back between the two hot water bottles and taken to the patient. Ask him to sit up for a moment so that the compress can be rolled from the back round the chest in such a way that one layer of material remains between the curd cheese and the skin. The towel holds it in place with the safety pins. The patient is covered with the bedclothes, but make sure that his shoulders are also tucked in.

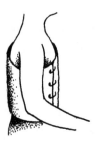

The compress should remain in place until it has dried out. If the patient says that it feels uncomfortable, the compress should be removed. The patient should then quickly put on his clothes. (It's a good idea to warm these up in advance.) He should rest for at least half an hour. The cloth is then rinsed with cold water in a bucket, which is emptied into the toilet.

This treatment can be given every day, or three times a week, depending on the complaint.

Another method is to apply the curd cheese or the cloth in such a way that the curd cheese is in direct contact with the skin.

(b) Breast compress

A curd cheese compress can be given for a breast infection (mastitis) after a woman has had a baby. In this case the compress is administered cold. This soothes the pain, and the sour substance dissipates the infection as it dries up.

REQUIREMENTS

— a cloth for the compress
— a container of curd cheese
— a spatula or spoon

PROCEDURE

Wash your hands. The cloth for the compress should first be ironed to eliminate the danger of infection. It is easy to cause more external infections through the nipples if the treatment is not performed hygienically.

Place the clean cloth on a towel and apply the curd cheese with a spatula or spoon, which should first be rinsed in hot water. The amount of curd cheese depends on the size of the breast and the inflammation. The compress should amply cover the area. When the curd cheese has been applied, all the edges are folded over and the compress is laid on the breast so that there is one layer of material between the curd cheese and the skin. Cover with a bra and top clothes.

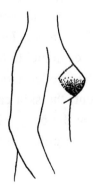

When the curd cheese has thoroughly dried out after twenty minutes, remove the compress and rinse the material in cold water.

NOTE: The compress must be removed after a maximum of twenty minutes to prevent it becoming warm and actually stimulating the inflammation.

This treatment can be given once or twice a day, and in serious or acute cases after every feed.

(c) Other inflammations

Other inflammations which can be treated with curd cheese include boils and acne. In the case of boils, it is slightly heated and applied in a small compress. Then wash your hands thoroughly.

Acne can be treated easily with a face mask. For this purpose, apply a thin layer of curd cheese to the face (for instance one to three times a week), leave to dry for about twenty minutes and then wash off with water.

7.2 Salt water wash

This treatment is aimed at regulating superfluous fluid processes in the human body. In coming into contact with the whole skin the limits of the body are felt more clearly. The clear structure of the salt acts as a kind of 'example' to the organism. The nervous system is formed from the ectoderm, or outer skin, at the embryonic stage of development; the skin can thus be described as a sensory organ. By bathing the body with salt the characteristics of the sensory system, as described in the first part of this book, are stimulated.

REQUIREMENTS

— a washbasin or bowl
— fine sea salt

— a bath thermometer
— a face flannel
— a measuring jug
— a towel

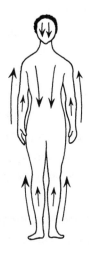

PROCEDURE

It is best to have the treatment in the morning, immediately on waking. The clothes to be worn after the treatment are laid out, and possibly warmed.

Fill the washbasin or bowl with water at 34°C (93°F). Use one level dessertspoonful (9g, 1/3 oz) of salt per litre (quart) of water, and dissolve in the measuring jug. Add this to the water. The bathroom (or other room) should be at a comfortable temperature. For every stroke, saturate the face flannel with salt water. Treat the body in the following order: face, arms with a few swift strokes down to the trunk, pat dry with the towel, then the back, with a few long movements down, pat dry, and finally the chest, again moving the flannel down to the waist. Dress the top half of the body.

The legs are also treated with a few swift movements upwards and then dried with the towel. Then get dressed. It is best not to have a rest after this treatment, but to go for a short walk.

7.3 Baths

(a) Oil baths

All the external treatments described in the preceding chapter are *localized* applications; in other words, something that is externally applied, on or around a particular area of the body. If the treatment involves a bath (full length bath), this is a *total* treatment. The doctor's advice is important in choosing the quality and type of treatment. This is always the case for an oil bath.

As treatment with an oil bath requires expert guidance, both from the therapeutic and the technical point of view, it is advisable to have this therapy in a therapy centre.

Nevertheless, for many people the distance to a centre will be too great for regular treatment. In consultation with the doctor, it is possible to find ways of treating the patient with oil baths to be given at home. A few general guidelines follow below.

REQUIREMENTS

    — a bathtub (for children, a baby bath or bowl)
    — bath thermometer
    — litre (quart) bottle with screw top
    — one teaspoon
    — oil
    — towelling bathrobe
    — towel

PROCEDURE

Shut the windows and make sure the room and the bathroom are comfortably warm. Place the towel on the pillow of the bed where the patient will rest after the treatment. Fold back the covers to the foot of the bed.

120

The bath is filled with water at body temperature (37°C, 98.6°F: use a bath thermometer). Fill the litre bottle with water at the same temperature and add three teaspoons of oil (for children in a small bath, two teaspoons is enough). Now shake the bottle for two or three minutes so that the oil is evenly distributed throughout the water. (Therapy centres have special equipment for this process which considerably enhances the effect of the treatment.) When it has been shaken, pour the bottle into the bath. The patient then gets in and lies as still as possible.

If the water cools down, it can be warmed up by holding the shower hose under water and slowly adding hot water. This should be done very carefully so that the distribution of oil in the water and the patient's perception of this is not disturbed. The temperature of the water can be adapted, depending on the individual, between 36° and 38°C (97° and 100.5°F).

These baths are prescribed by the doctor as a cure. The bath should be given regularly once, or at most twice, a week, always on the same day and at the same time.

The duration of treatment increases progressively. Thus, you begin with five minutes, the second bath takes seven, and the third bath takes twelve minutes; for children, the treatment can last a maximum of fifteen minutes, and for adults a maximum of twenty minutes. Never leave the patient alone in the bath.

When the time is up, the patient gets out of the bath. He is not dried, but puts on a bathrobe straightaway and lies down in bed. The towel is placed round his head and over his shoulders and he is warmly tucked up, making sure the shoulders are covered. He now rests for at least half an hour, or better still, for a whole hour. The curtains should be drawn and all sounds avoided as far as possible.

During his rest the patient will soon notice an intense feeling of warmth permeating him. This feeling can continue for a long time, sometimes a few days. Try to 'save' this feeling and retain it as much as possible with warm clothes on the one hand, and on the other hand, by leaving the upper parts of the body 'cool' in a healthy way. Therefore avoid excessive sensory stimuli, for example, radio and television.

The thin layer of oil, which remains on the skin stays there for quite a long time. To retain this effect it is better not to have a bath or shower for twenty-four hours after the oil bath.

NOTE: A thyme oil bath for children with asthma and bronchitis is often an effective treatment for restoring the lack of harmony in the air and water organism in the central area.

Sometimes it is difficult to keep a child quiet in the bath for the indicated period. A small boat or toy fish will usually help to pass the time, but animals or boats, which are wound up, are certainly not advisable in this situation as they can completely destroy the therapeutic process. While the child is resting it is a good idea to tell him a story or read him a fairy-tale. If this is done carefully, he will certainly rest and this enhances the effect of the whole treatment.

(b) 'Substance' baths

It may have become apparent that in almost every form of treatment *water* plays an important role. The water element brings life and joins heaven and earth; water vapour rises to unknown heights and returns to earth in the form of raindrops. It is constantly changing form in this cycle.

In antiquity and even now, water is important in many religious activities, for example, washing the feet before entering a temple, or in baptisms. It is a mediating substance in human life. Therefore, it is understandable that for therapeutic purposes it also forms an essential link in the healing process.

In addition, it contains many other possibilities, which are used in giving a 'substance' bath: in fact, it can assimilate virtually any matter. In a 'substance' bath something is added to the water in order to surround the whole of the person in a watery environment. These substances can be bath milks, different sorts of tea, and minerals, (salts, soda) as well as milk, egg, lemon and honey, as in the so-called nourishing bath.

REQUIREMENTS

  — bathtub (for children a baby bath or bowl)
  — bath thermometer
  — measuring jug
  — towelling bathrobe
  — towel

PROCEDURE

Make sure that the room is comfortably warm. Run the bath with water at 37°C (98.6°F). At this temperature human life processes take place. The following technique can be used to restore some of the natural movement to the water, which has passed many purification plants, gone through many channels and pipes, and been stored in a tanks for a long time. With one hand, make a slow movement describing the figure eight through the water (lemniscate). The movement should be rounded and carried out

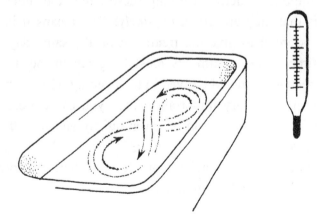

rhythmically. Keep this up until you feel that the water is actually 'following' your hand. Then add the substance, and the patient can get into the bath.

The water should now be moved as little as possible. If necessary, add hot water to keep it at the right temperature. The treatment is complete after fifteen to twenty minutes and the patient can get out of the bath. He is not dried off, but puts on his bathrobe immediately and lies down in bed. A towel is placed over his head and he is tucked up warmly with the rest of the bedclothes, making sure the shoulders are covered. Then he has a rest or sleep.

During this rest the patient will quickly feel that he is surrounded by a comfortable warmth and will feel relaxed. (Prevent perspiration.) After the rest, the skin should be completely dried and he should wear warm clothes.

Baths of rosemary and lavender can easily be taken at home, especially immediately on waking or before going to bed at night. Rosemary produces a refreshing 'awake' feeling, and it is understandable that it is best not to have a rest after this treatment, but to go for a short walk. A lavender bath has a relaxing effect, and if it is taken in the evening, it will induce a peaceful sleep.

An important factor in giving these baths and other treatment is that they are given *regularly*. This means it is absolutely essential to give the treatment on the same day at the same time. Some treatments must be given in the morning; other treatments must be given in the evening. However, if the time is of secondary importance, then you can choose when you feel the treatment can be given quietly and with the least disturbance.

Rhythm is an inherent part of life, and therefore forms an essential link in the healing process.

7.4 Rubbing the whole body

After a long period of physical or psychological illness, one way of helping the organism to recover is by rubbing the whole body with skin tone lotion to stimulate the life forces.

REQUIREMENTS

    — two sheets
    — a large towel
    — two hot water bottles
    — skin tonic
    — bowl

PROCEDURE

The room and the bed are prepared. Shut the windows and make sure that the temperature is comfortable. Clear the bedside table and warm the bottle of skin tonic in the bowl of hot water. The patient should go to the toilet and the curtains are drawn. Wash your hands. Place the large towel over the pillow and the two sheets (if possible, use flannel sheets) across the bed, one at the head and one at the foot, so that they overlap in the middle.

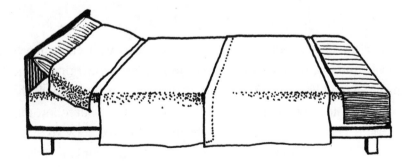

The hot water bottles are placed at the foot of the bed. The patient undresses, keeping on his underpants. He sits down on the bed.

Shake some skin tone lotion onto the hand and make some calm, rhythmic, repeated movements over the back, keeping the hands next to each other so that you are stroking parallel to the spinal column from the top down. Never stroke over the spinal column. Do not use too much skin tone lotion as this produces a sticky feeling and clogs up the skin. When the lotion has been rubbed into the back, the patient lies down. Put a little more lotion on the hand and rub the arms, rubbing towards the heart — towards the shoulders, with calm, rhythmic, repeated movements. When you have done one arm, cover it with a sheet and then do the other arm.

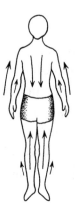

For the chest, take a little more lotion, and with calm movements, rub from the shoulders down to the navel a few times. The hands should be next to each other and move symmetrically. If the patient's rate of breathing is normal, the movements can follow this rhythm. Then tuck up the rest of the top half of the body so that a fold of the sheet comes between the arms and the trunk, and there is no skin touching skin. The towel is placed round the head.

The legs are treated with the same movements, rubbing upwards towards the heart. First do one leg and cover it up, then the other leg and cover it up. Finally, do a few gentle but fairly firm strokes along the soles of the feet and then cover these up too. Place the hot water bottles on either side. Tuck the patient up with a blanket or duvet. If possible, the patient should be left in this 'package' for at least twenty minutes, better still for thirty or forty minutes. If he falls asleep, he can remain wrapped up until he wakes. It is best to give this treatment before the afternoon nap, unless the doctor suggests another time.

In any case, *rest* during the treatment is extremely important — avoid all sensory impressions, as this disturbs the processes of perception when the patient is wrapped up. After the treatment and the rest period it is important that the patient dresses warmly so that he can retain the warmth resulting from the treatment for as long as possible.

7.5 Foot-baths

Foot-baths can be given for various reasons: to stimulate the circulation, to draw trapped metabolic process away from the head, or to treat the skin of the feet and lower legs.

(a) Alternating foot-bath

REQUIREMENTS

- two foot-baths
- a towel
- a bath thermometer
- a watch

PROCEDURE

The foot-baths are placed in the bathtub or shower, or on the floor on top of a bath mat. Place a chair next to the foot-bath. The foot-bath should be large enough for the patient's feet to fit in comfortably in a normal position, and so that the edge of the foot-bath reaches up to the knee.

One foot-bath is filled two-thirds full of water at 38°C (100°F), and the other also two-thirds full of water at 20°C (68°F). Use a bath thermometer. The patient bares the lower legs to above the knees, making sure that his trouser legs are not constricting, and places the legs in the warm foot-bath for two or three minutes. Make sure that his shoulders are warmly covered. Then immediately transfer the feet for one minute into the cold foot-bath, and then back to the warm foot-bath for two or three minutes. Alternate in this way three or four times, ending with the warm bath. (If necessary, top up with hot water.)

The whole treatment should last about fifteen minutes. Then the feet and legs are thoroughly dried and the patient puts on a pair of knee length stockings. It is better to give this treatment in the evening before going to bed, so that it is immediately followed by a rest.

(b) Mustard foot-bath

See Section 6.7 (d).

(c) Foot-bath with medication

REQUIREMENTS

- — one foot-bath
- — prescribed medication
- — if necessary, a measuring jug

— if necessary, bandages
— a towel
— a bath thermometer

PROCEDURE

The foot-bath (for size, see above) is put out and filled two-thirds full with water at 37°C (98.6°F) unless otherwise prescribed. The prescribed quantity of medication is added and stirred into the water with a few gentle movements.

The patient bares the lower legs to above the knees and wears warm clothes on the upper half of his body. The legs are placed in the foot-bath. Cover the patient's knees with a towel so that it also covers the foot-bath. See that the patient remains as relaxed as possible during the treatment. The treatment does not usually last more than fifteen to twenty minutes. Keep the water at the right temperature by adding warm water from time to time.

After the treatment, pat the feet and legs dry. If necessary, bandage them up, and if possible, the patient then wears knee-length stockings.

7.6 Poultice

A poultice is given if it is not possible to rub (or massage) the patient, because of the nature of the complaint (burns, inflammations).

REQUIREMENTS

— a smooth piece of material (cotton)
— lint or flannel
— ointment

— a spatula or spoon
— a wooden board
— a bandage
— a plaster
— a towel

PROCEDURE

The part of the body to be treated is bared and the towel is laid under it to protect the bedding. Wash the hands thoroughly. The piece of cotton should be cut to size and ironed, and should not be frayed around the edges. Gauze should not be used for this treatment, as the fabric adheres to any wound very easily. The cloth is placed on the clean wooden board or plate, and the ointment is spread on to the middle of the cloth with the spatula or the handle of the spoon. The plate or board acts as a hard background which makes it easier to spread out the ointment.

Hold the cloth by the edge and put it in place. Cover with the lint or flannel, which should cover the poultice completely and should therefore be slightly larger. Use a bandage or surgical bandage to keep the poultice in place, and, if necessary, stick down with a piece of plaster.

The doctor will indicate how often this treatment should be given. For poultices using calendula, arnica and combudoron (see Chapter 6). For this treatment always use clean materials because of the danger of infection.

In some cases poultices with metallic ointments are prescribed. These can be used a few times in succession. Just add a little bit of ointment onto the same cloth.

III

Birth, Illness and Death

8. Pregnancy and Birth

8.1 Pregnancy

Although a chapter on pregnancy and birth does not really belong in a book about the sick, we would like to include some guidelines so that this joyful time can be experienced as positively and consciously as possible.

In Chapter 2, we showed that man develops through repeated lives on earth. From this point of view it is interesting to note that pregnancy can be seen as more than a chance event. We can think of the child making a decision in another world, seeking the parents who will make it possible for him to develop in the way he wants to develop. Following this line of thought, we can clearly feel the responsibility that we have as parents. The child could not have come to other parents as easily: it came to us.

A mother may feel a warm sense of gratitude and joy that this new arrival has chosen her. It is certainly worthwhile allowing this inner warmth to suffuse her again and again, remembering constantly that someone really wished to come to her. This will make it less difficult on the days where she might be inclined to a more miserable outlook. It will make it easier to accept that she has to give up or change some habits.

(a) Rhythm in daily life

Undoubtedly, there will be various habits, which an expectant mother will have to change, or perhaps it is better to say that she will wish to change them. During pregnancy it is a good idea to try and divide the day up into a regular and rhythmic pattern. It is important to discover times of rest during the day, as this will also be of benefit to the development of the child. In addition, it prepares her for the most important thing of all, the rhythm that must be established once the child is born.

The mother will discover for herself that it is best to avoid carrying heavy weights, standing for long periods of time or bending over a lot during pregnancy. After a violent shock or strong emotions anyone may have a sense of not being at one with their body. During pregnancy this feeling is intensified, and in this situation, it is good to try and stand back from what has happened, not letting emotions take over. It can be a help to listen to some beautiful music, or to look at a work of art, like a reproduction of Raphael's *Sistine Madonna*.

(b) Nutrition

Obviously it is important to stop smoking and drinking alcohol. Try to drink as little coffee and tea, as possible, and eat less meat. These products with their strong connection to the earth, do not help the child who is still in another world, and needs to be brought very slowly to earth. Various herbal teas are good alternatives for coffee and tea. A daily dessertspoonful of honey is almost cosmic food.

In consultation with a doctor or midwife, calcium salts I and II (Weleda) can be taken from the beginning of pregnancy.

It sometimes happens, especially at the *beginning* of pregnancy, that mothers to be have an almost unnatural desire for strong flavours, exotic or unusual foods. In many cases, they will bolt this down, as if they expect to be caught in the act. The body, which previously belonged to her alone, is now shared with another. This is not a pleasant experience, and she is inclined

134

to reach for something familiar and supportive, something that has a specific sour or salty taste. If she can recognize this, she may succeed in controlling these cravings and finding a more balanced diet. For example, some muesli for breakfast, sour fruits throughout the day, and crisp salad with the evening meal. During the first months avoid too many carbohydrates, as these make you unnecessarily fat.

AFTER ABOUT THREE MONTHS, the mother will be more comfortable with the pregnancy. This will be accompanied by inner peace, making her feel more settled and self-confident. She will no longer feel the need for sour food and will increasingly prefer sweet things. Try not to keep reaching for the biscuit tin, but opt for sweet-tasting fruit or unsalted almonds. Eat a lot of green vegetables during this time, for the leaf is the part of the plant that forms the equilibrium between the root and the flower, relating particularly to the rhythmic elements in the body (see Chapter 3).

DURING THE LAST FEW MONTHS, the child grows considerably. It is better not to eat too many vegetables, such as brassicas, leeks and onions as these might lead to stomach cramps. Eat regular freshly-prepared meals containing cereals and in order to activate the intestines gently, drink fruit juice every day. It is important to eat regularly, and it is better to have several small meals a day than to consume large quantities at few sittings.

Make sure your bowels move regularly, and if necessary, drink some linseed in water every morning (the evening before, leave a dessertspoonful of linseed to soak).

During the last month it often happens that there is a heavy, pressing feeling in the lower abdomen. In this case it is soothing to sit in a bath with some lime blossom tea. A bath or tub should be one-third filled with water at about 37°C (99°F) and the infusion of 10 g (under $^1/_2$ oz) of lime blossom has a relaxing effect. Make sure that the water does not cool down too much.

135

Detailed advice about physical care and exercises for pregnancy are beyond the scope of this little book. If you wish to do special exercises for pregnancy, contact existing groups, for example, ante-natal classes at the local maternity hospital or health centre.

8.2 Birth and confinement

In some cases it happens that a child is 'too late,' or at least later than it was calculated, and the doctor or midwife may suggest that it will have to be induced. For many parents this is a very frightening idea, for they have quite a different image of a peaceful birth. Unless there are other abnormalities, the doctor or midwife will probably agree if you ask for two more days' delay. Try to be as calm as possible during those two days, enjoy beautiful things and allow yourself to relax as much as possible. Don't start ironing piles of washing or cleaning out cupboards. In this way you give the child a sign that it is welcome; you're saying, 'If it's time to come, come now.' Very often the child will be born normally if this advice is followed. Try to give birth without any anaesthetic, unless this is medically essential, so that you can experience the arrival of your child consciously. It is good for the father, or another person close to the child, to be present at the birth. Make sure that the room is as peaceful and comforting as possible. There should be no clutter, but it shouldn't be a cold, sterile place. The child wants to come *home*.

The chance of very heavy bleeding is reduced if the mother has five drops of arnica D6 dissolved in a little water every three hours for the first twenty-four hours after the birth.

(a) Breastfeeding

In order to stimulate breastfeeding the child is put to the mother's breast soon after it is born. The sucking reflex is very strong for the first twenty to forty minutes after the birth. As a reaction to the sucking the uterus contracts strongly.

If the nipples have been regularly bathed with lemon juice from the fourth or fifth month of pregnancy, they will not be painful during feeding.

If feeding proves difficult, it is a good idea to drink about a litre of barley water every day (see end of Section 5.3). The drink is made from polished barley. It is useful to know that cauliflower also stimulates lactation, as does aniseed. If none of this works, you can still try the Weleda lactagogue tea, perhaps after consulting your doctor or midwife. The other extreme is when there is too much milk leading to hard, painful areas. In this case a curd compress is soothing (see Section 7.1 (b)).

For the first fortnight note the times when the baby wakes up and is fed. Often a pattern emerges, which may be the rhythm of your child. Though of course he should not be fed on demand every time, it is a good starting point to really listen for a fortnight and then use this to draw up a permanent timetable.

(b) The cradle

The cradle must be ready for the birth. It is best surrounded by a large curtain, preferably of plain material, for example, apricot-coloured or pink, covered by another that is light blue. This is better than a material printed with a motif such as dolls or teddy bears. Make sure that the cradle is warmed up. It is vital to ensure that the child comes to earth slowly, so he should not be removed from the mother immediately. Ask the doctor or midwife if the baby can be put on the mother's stomach before the umbilical cord is cut. This can be a very important moment for both mother and child.

137

Before dressing the baby warmly he must be carefully dabbed clean all over. It is best not to bathe him allowing the protective and nutritional layer on his skin to be retained. He should be dressed in a thin woollen vest covered with a woollen jumper. In the beginning use soft cotton nappies (diapers). (If they are washed and rinsed thoroughly a few times in advance, they will lose their stiffness) A thick pair of lambs-wool pants helps to prevent the cradle from becoming wet, making plastic pants superfluous. A warm flannel cloth wrapped around the abdomen and legs protects the child from cold and gives it the swaddling it needs.

(c) The first few weeks

It is not necessary to bath the baby every day. Obviously it is important to make sure that it is clean when changing a dirty nappy. When the baby is given a bath, make sure the room is pleasantly warm, the bath water is at body temperature (37°C, 98.6°F) and the towel and clothes are warmed in advance. The differences in temperature should not be too great.

Do not take the baby outside straightaway. For the first three weeks it is enough to place the warm cradle by an open window for ten or fifteen minutes every day. Make sure that the head does not get too cold. The baby should wear a thin silk or cotton cap, even in summer, unless he has a great head of hair, which will act as natural protection.

If you go for a walk, try to go to a park or wood as quickly as possible, as a busy shopping street is a terrible place for a baby. You actually force the baby to hear and see everything that is happening in our noisy outside world. The baby doesn't have to 'wake up' to this so quickly, so leave it in the warm, safe, enclosed baby world as long as possible.

9. Sleep

Our lives are full of rhythms, such as the four changing seasons, the twelve months of the year and the seven days of the week. There are also the rhythms mentioned earlier, such as heartbeat and breathing, and the 'rhythm' in the structure of our vertebrae. Because it is an inherent part of life, many therapies are given in a rhythmic manner. Water in therapeutic baths is moved rhythmically, and homoeopathic medicines are prepared in rhythmic processes.

One of the rhythms of our daily lives is the change from day to night, waking and sleeping. Before going into possible remedies for sleeping problems, we shall look at sleep itself.

When we are asleep, we are incapable of thought and are not conscious of our surroundings in any way; we only rediscover them when we wake up in the morning. We also lose our sense of time; for example, we may wake up after an hour feeling that we have slept all night. Our self and our senses are active in a different way from when we are awake. While our life forces remain linked to our physical body during sleep (all the biological processes such as respiration, circulation and digestion continue to function), our consciousness, the part of us which makes us a real individual in life — that is the Self and the perceiving soul — remain intensely bound up with the spiritual world at night.

As we saw in Chapter 2, our Self and our soul combine in the physical and ethereal body (life force body) when we are awake, and we are able to live as conscious individuals. After a period of combining in this way the Self and the soul relax and expand into the spiritual world; this is the moment at which we fall asleep. (Many people have a sense of floating or flying at this moment, and this can be seen as an image of the soul and self moving into the spiritual world.) When we wake up after a healthy night's sleep we feel refreshed and rested because the soul and the self can combine with the body once again with renewed strength from the spiritual world. Many people wake up with a new idea or a thought, which sheds new light on a particular situation. For example, the great creative genius, Raphael, saw one of his unfinished Madonna paintings completed before him when he woke up. Musicians such as Bruckner and Schubert sometimes woke up with new melodies in their head. Russian fairy-tales express this in the recurring phrase: 'The morning is wiser than the evening.'

To sleep really well a person must therefore be able to let go, he must step back and be able to relax. If he has difficulties or problems, the process of letting go will be more difficult, because thoughts and feelings will become involved, taking possession of him just before he goes to sleep. Of course, illness or pain may be the reason why the process of letting go does not occur. In this case, medical help is necessary. However, if this is not the case, it is a good idea to take a look at our life and see what we could change in it, and how its rhythm may be strengthened.

In the first place, if you cannot sleep, there is no need to panic, because it does not matter if you miss a night's sleep. As people get older, they tend to sleep less soundly. This should be accepted, and if necessary, they should stop having a midday nap so that they sleep well at night, or perhaps start having a midday nap so that they can create a new rhythm. This differs from person to person.

Children also have periods of sleeping badly and being afraid. This is often a time when they experience the gradual loss of the safe world of childhood, resulting in a feeling of loneliness or being abandoned. Questions like: 'Mum, how would I find you if I died?' are indicative of a child's mood. In such cases it is important to stay with the child, accept his fears and not brush them aside. When children are scared, it may be necessary to take a look under the bed with them, or look in dark corners. It can also be helpful to tell a story or talk together about what has happened. Finally, a night light or leaving the door ajar can restore the child's confidence.

On the other hand, adults have to find a way themselves of coping with sleepless hours. Is it best to lie down and think about things, or does this lead to even greater restlessness as a result of chaotic thoughts? Do you stay in bed tossing and turning, or do you get up after lying in bed for an hour to make a hot drink or read for a little? Reading relaxing literature can be helpful to step back from certain thoughts or feelings and concentrate on others.

Lying in late in the morning is no solution for sleeping problems. Often the problem of not sleeping well disappears by itself when the person or child concerned is confident that he will be able to sleep. Avoid starting to take sleeping pills because you can become accustomed, or even addicted, to them, and this can permanently disturb the natural process.

When the sleeping and waking rhythm is disrupted in seriously ill patients, other factors sometimes play a role and it may be necessary for them to take medicines which make it possible for them to derive new strength from the spiritual world, or to re-establish a health-giving rhythm between waking and sleeping. Obviously a natural product is always preferable. In addition, it may be helpful for the sick to keep the normal going to bed 'ritual' unchanged as far as possible. When they go to bed many people have a fixed pattern of habit, which gives them a sense of security. Because sick people are dependent on others, this fixed pattern is often disturbed, and this can make getting to sleep difficult.

There are many remedies, which can help a healthy person to prepare for the night. For example, you could go for a short stroll in the evening, for fresh air has a relaxing effect and stimulates the circulation. You could drink a cup of warm (aniseed-flavoured) milk instead of coffee (caffeine) or tea (tannin). It is obviously not a good idea to have a large meal before going to sleep, though if you are hungry you could have a snack. While it is not advisable to watch television late at night, pore over the newspaper, or study, some people find literature with a religious or spiritual content relaxing, and others find that fairy-tales make good bedtime reading. The essential thing is that you direct your thoughts at the content of what you are reading, and in this way stand back from the daily grind of life: a sort of inner orientation.

In addition to these normal routines, it may be helpful to have a lavender foot-bath: warm water (38°C, 98.6°F). with a tablespoonful of lavender bath essence for every bucket of water (see Section 7.5). A cup of warm herbal tea is also often helpful, such as lemon balm, hops, camomile, passion flower or valerian. By experimenting, find out which works best.

In addition to a tranquil environment without disturbing light or sound, a warm and comfortable bed with a good mattress, and being completely relaxed, the way in which you inwardly prepare for the night is also very important. For many people it is helpful to say a prayer or a meaningful verse. It also helps to imagine the starry night sky and concentrate on the thought of a particular prayer, mantra or meditation; the self and the soul are better able to free themselves of the earth.[4]

Rudolf Steiner wrote various verses for children and adults to say at night and in the morning to accompany waking and sleeping. Various images can also be helpful for the soul to relinquish the day, such as imagining how a rose loses its petals one by one, or counting sheep as they cross a bridge. In addition, Rudolf Steiner suggested an evening exercise for those who wish to undergo inner training, consisting of thinking back through all the events of the day, but in reverse order. In this way you observe yourself without experiencing the emotions again. It is a peaceful way of rounding off the day.

An evening prayer or text is not only a beneficial activity for those who are sick or for people who have problems getting to sleep, it is also a good way for healthy people to go into the night.

In order to enjoy a good night's rest you must always attempt to be wide 'awake' in every aspect throughout the day. Obviously being awake during the day starts with waking up properly in the morning. For in order to function well, it is important to create a balance in a disturbed rhythm of sleeping and waking in a natural way. It is only then that you can come properly to yourself, and join harmoniously in the great cosmic rhythm.

10. Sickness and Destiny

Whenever anyone is sick, the question arises: how did I get this illness? When it is a simple cold, it is a relief to remember the moment that one 'caught cold,' or who 'passed it on.' However, when it is a more serious illness, the question becomes more significant, and the 'why?' or 'why *me?*' can be important. A sense of impotence and insecurity often takes over when you have to change the pattern of your daily life for the sick bed, and move from a vertical to a horizontal position.

The sense of dependence and feeling beholden will result in a situation of crisis, quite apart from the sickness itself. This can become all the more momentous as the illness lasts longer, or appears to be of a more serious nature. If the illness is seen only as a disturbance in the pattern of daily life, it is difficult not to be rebellious or fall into a state of lethargy. But it is also possible to wonder: What does this illness want of me? Why has it come upon me at this stage of my life and in this place? What can I do with it? Could this sickness have a purpose? What is happening in my life?

As fellow human beings, we are able to create the space in which these questions, which are often buried and hidden, can be heard by the patient himself. It is therefore a good idea to make sure that the patient is really not disturbed at certain times of day.

It is possible that we are present at one of the most important moments in someone's development precisely because daily life is not dominating the real meaning. Many people feel thrown back on their own resources, but empty-handed. When we take a careful look at illness, we sometimes recognize a great conflict between our thoughts, feelings and impulses to act, on the one hand, and the body, which has given up, on the other. In fact, there is a conflict between the inside and the outside world, for to some extent the body is the outside world to the human soul.

It is, therefore, extremely important that attention is paid to proper sleep; if possible, for seven or eight hours from two hours before midnight to the next morning, so that the patient can build up new strength for the next day from the world of sleep. Problems in life, which are taken into sleep, can be seen in a new light as the result of an encounter between man's inner world and the world of sleep.

Many people are familiar with the feeling of waking up with an idea or a solution to a particular problem. Sometimes the problem itself has changed and looks different the next day. Why is this the case? The study of anthroposophy gives the answer that the world where the human soul resides during sleep is a spiritual world where man lives unconsciously, and where he is receptive to new strength and new impulses. It is the same world that he came from before birth, and where he goes after death.

Our physical body has its limitations within one earth life. We are bound to a particular model with its own boundaries. However, man's inner soul is not completely bound to these limitations, and it is particularly during illness that it is able to recognize some of its own destiny and possibly develop new initiatives, or give a new meaning to life. Thus the sickness can become a blessing. The patient can contribute freely and actively to his recovery in an important way, so that he becomes a different person through this recovery.

In this case the illness has helped to reveal something. Something is healed and there is a new harmony resulting from the encounter with the forces of the higher self, which is the core of man's inner being; a recognition of his own inner quality, usually hidden behind a veil. There is a vision of a new direction in life. Only when this occurs can it be said that healing has really taken place. A condition for this is that the patient is surrounded by a therapeutic environment, in which he is treated with warmth and concern.

If it is not possible to restore the lack of harmony, which exists during the sickness, the patient will die. The new forces from the spiritual world, which join us to our physical bodies in the morning after sleep, are unable to connect with the physical body and finally fail altogether, if the instrument is too damaged. The result is death, and man enters a new stage of his existence.

After death a new phase of development starts in the spiritual world, which is completely different from that on earth. This is a process in which the fruits of life are assimilated and adapted, gradually leading man to a new incarnation on earth.

A man's experiences during his lifetime, the strength with which a sick person has borne and accepted his lot, are adapted after death to form the seed for the next life. Thus, an active and positive attitude during illness will produce a strong seed. The will to experience the pain and not to resort to painkillers immediately, is equivalent to an investment in the processes that follow death. This is reflected in the spiritual world, and from a higher insight it acts as a stimulus for the preparation of a new life.

One takes a sort of 'extract' of life to the next life on earth, which is not a repetition, but another step in the development of the individual. Just as we receive strength for the next day from sleep, we also receive strength for our next life on earth between death and rebirth. The newborn child comes from a previous existence; he does not arrive in the world as a *tabula rasa*.

In this way, both cure and death can be considered as steps in man's development; they both have a profound meaning and significance. Sickness is a key which shows us things about ourselves, if we have the courage to ask the question: what can this sickness tell me about my life?

11. Nursing the Critically and Terminally Ill

Nursing a patient through the last stage of his life is often a difficult task because it confronts us with our own insecurity. It takes courage for us to find the peace within ourselves, which we need to approach the patient. He often has many unspoken questions and we are constantly faced with the feeling day after day: 'Should I try — no matter how unsure I am — to answer this unspoken question, should I wait, and then what should I say?'

If we constantly carry this insecurity around with us, it often leads to remorse or guilt because we think we have failed somewhere. If, on the other hand, we have faith and respect for the destiny of the other person, and we support him with warmth, it is possible to conquer our insecurity, and in this way develop a positive attitude towards the process of dying. The patient will feel this response as a confirmation.

People who are at the end of their life may pass through different stages, as described by Elisabeth Kübler-Ross: denial, anger, rationalization, depression and acceptance. We can constantly try to respond to these moods with tenderness. We must learn to view them objectively, as part of the process, and not feel personally affected if the patient is unreasonable or unjust. Sometimes one can feel that he has never been like that before, and it seems as though he is being subjected to a power greater than himself.

Most probably a great deal more happens in the person's soul during this decisive stage than we can perceive. The only correct response to this is to surround the patient with warmth and patience, and especially to try not to be hurt and irritated.

For example, if the patient becomes restless, and obviously at a stage where he finds it difficult to cope with this restlessness, it is possible to help him with nursing techniques by providing him with an environment in which he can find a sort of balance and support for his inner restlessness. Make sure that the room is tidy in every respect. This includes looking after the flowers and removing nursing aids, such as head supports and a blanket arch from the room, as well as extra pillows and blankets. The waste-paper basket should be empty. Make sure that the patient is tucked up, and if he tosses and turns, give him a warm nightshirt or pyjamas and bed-socks. In addition, if the patient and the other members of the family do not mind, a sense of extra security can be obtained by surrounding the bed with rails, and covering these with rugs or blankets. In this way the patient will not hurt himself and it provides extra protection. (In some cases the rails can be used only at night.) Sometimes he must be left alone. Possibly he is still able to sit up in a chair with armrests. This will tire him, so that he will fall asleep afterwards and be freed of his restlessness for a while.

Nursing is an art. Try to use your imagination to discover what will be comfortable for the patient. Stay near him as much as possible, or at least within earshot, and make sure that he can always reach a bell.

When the patient groans and you ask if he feels pain, it is not always so. During the last stages he will often feel less pain. It would be wrong to give painkillers in this case and tranquillizers should also be avoided as much as possible — obviously unless the patient requests them. Consciousness is impaired by these substances, and we should try to prevent this and allow the person to be himself for as long as possible.

In the final days the patient should still be washed as usual and the bed should be made every day. In this way he retains his independence for as long as possible. Obviously, he should still be taking enough fluids. (Remember that one teaspoonful of fluid is very little; there are one hundred and twenty teaspoonfuls of water in one glass.)

Great care should be taken to ensure proper nursing so that there will be no complications: caring for the mouth, wetting the lips, preventing bedsores, turning the patient, rubbing. Every patient will need different nursing care, but above all our own inner attitude will be a great support. In every situation one will have to assess whether the patient wants someone around, or wants to be alone for a while. However, never abandon him. Try to be aware of what you say to him at the right moment, and remember that at all stages the patient will continue to hope; allow this hope to be, but do not raise false hopes.

It is important to wait and see what the patient wishes to achieve in his discussion. This sometimes conflicts completely with a conversation which took place just before. Experience has shown that it is best to start with an open-ended question, for example, a remark about something in the room. The patient's mood can be gauged from his answer and tone of voice; you can tell whether he is afraid or feels the need to talk about something else. The patient has a right to the possibility of changing the subject.

The important thing is to approach the patient with our whole being, listening intently to try and understand him. The atmosphere we create is based on our fundamental attitude. It is also the condition for a situation in which the patient can feel protected, and where the process of dying can take place unhampered.

Reading to a patient, from a book which he wishes to hear, which is familiar to him or he may have read before, can also be helpful in preparing for death, if he is ready for this. The Bible, a poem or a proverb, perhaps even one of the many lectures by Rudolf Steiner about life and death, can be a great support and help to combat fear.

If the patient feels the need to talk to a minister or priest, this should certainly be possible. Together they can discuss whether the patient wishes to receive the last rites. A calm discussion with the doctor or nurse about the way in which the final stages of illness will run its course, can be of great help. Always make sure that there is time for him to come to terms with things between these conversations or readings.

It is always advisable to nurse the patient at home unless the medical treatment required (and desired) makes this absolutely impossible. At home one is not bound by the organization, which is unavoidable in a hospital or nursing home, no matter how good the care. The patient's links with his own home are so important and his needs can be met so much more flexibly that everything possible should be done to enable him to stay at home.

There is often a problem in getting enough help. If friends or acquaintances offer to lend a hand, it can be a great help if they do the shopping or come and stay the night. They could also read to the patient or simply be near to give other members of the household a chance to retire.

As death approaches, the patient may have fewer complaints, feel like doing all sorts of things and start to make plans. He may experience a general feeling of well-being (euphoria), which is actually in conflict with the gravity of the situation. In this situation, when he feels less acutely, great care should be taken not to make hot water bottles too hot. Painkillers, which may have been used, may no longer be necessary.

Subsequently, the patient's sight deteriorates, and then the voluntary and involuntary muscles become weaker; a patient who was not incontinent may become so. His expression will change, and towards the end his pulse and breathing will slow down and become irregular. Remember that his hearing remains unimpaired for a long time, and you should not whisper or talk softly in the hall outside his room.

150

Throughout the whole nursing process wordless contact is of real importance. A single look or gesture, an encouraging pat on the hand can be very meaningful. It is not always necessary to talk, and talk may in fact be very tiring for the patient. It is much more important to listen, trying to understand and respond to the dying patient's wishes.

It can be difficult to determine the exact moment of death. But around this time one of the close relatives may wish to say something or lead a prayer.

When the patient has died, a number of things should be done. The time must be noted, and if the doctor is not present, he should be notified so that he can come and confirm the death. The deceased should be laid out flat, his eyes should be shut and a piece of damp cotton wool placed on the eyes. False teeth should be put back in the mouth. Shut the mouth by placing a rolled-up towel under the chin and a small pillow under the head. Remove or put on jewellery, after consulting with the relatives. Cross the deceased's hands. Lay out clean pyjamas or a night-dress, cut open down the back if necessary. Never use safety pins. Turn off the heating.

Nowadays, it is usual for the undertaker to deal with the last offices (a nurse will do so only in exceptional cases). In case the relatives prefer to do this themselves, we include a few guidelines (preferably carried out within two or three hours of death, and always with two people).

Get ready what is needed: a bowl of water, flannel and soap, towel; oiled cotton wool, surgical gauze, comb, nail-clippers, shaving things if necessary; clean linen and a rubber sheet to protect the sheets. When you have washed all that is necessary, protect the sheets and fill up the rectum with oiled cotton wool or surgical gauze. Cover the opening of the bladder as there is a possibility of urine leaking. Provide a clean sheet. Comb the

III. BIRTH, ILLNESS AND DEATH

deceased's hair and trim the nails. Then place a clean sheet over the deceased with his hands folded on top of it; the hands express an essential part of a person's nature. The sheet can have several folds so that it is not stretched taut, and single flowers can be placed in these folds. This counteracts the cold whiteness of the sheet surrounding the deceased with flowers. The flowers lying on the bed will wilt, and this reflects the gradual fading of the body and the separation of the soul.

When all this has been done, different ways can be used to enhance the atmosphere in the room where the deceased is lying with candles, flowers and so on. If possible, place candles on both sides so that no shadows fall on the face. There should be one or two chairs for those who wish to spend some time with the deceased. Perhaps good friends would like to watch over him for an hour or two in the night. If it was the wish of the deceased, one of the Gospels could be read, perhaps the Gospel of St John, or something, which was well loved by the deceased. If circumstances permit, it is good to leave the deceased in his own surroundings until the day of the interment or cremation.

Many who have crossed this threshold in near-death experiences have spoken about entering a world of light. An awareness of this world and a trust in it can act as a guide in caring for those who are dying.

Remedies to Keep at Home

A number of medicines and materials were mentioned in this book, which you will need to carry out treatments. These are available from a chemist, pharmacist or health shop. Below we provide a survey with some additional remedies. Weleda and Wala are the names of two companies which are concerned with producing specifically anthroposophical medicines. Their products are made from pure natural ingredients and according to rhythmic processes.

— Arnica ointment (Weleda) for bumps and bruises, and for use in the aftercare of bruising.

— Arnica lotion (Weleda).

— Combudoron ointment (Weleda) for small burns and the use in aftercare of larger burns, sunburn and insect bites.

— Calendula ointment (Weleda) for infected wounds and skin irritations.

— Calendula lotion (Weleda).

— Carbo betulae D3 tablets (Weleda) for digestive complaints (2–3 tablets every 1–2 hours. In acute cases, five tablets at a time.)

— Clairo (Weleda) for constipation. Do not make it too strong as this leads to cramp.

— Skin tone lotion (Weleda) to prevent bedsores.

— Cold and throat mixture (drops from Weleda) for flu; in acute cases, 10 drops in water every 2 hours, otherwise 15 drops three times a day.

— Massage oil (Weleda) or Carob oil for rubbing in case of muscular pain and cold painful limbs.

— Melissa comp. drops (Weleda). Use externally for head-aches, patting on the forehead, or internally for nausea, shock, emotional disturbance and fainting. 10 drops in some water or sugar.

— Sage pastels (Salvia from Wala) for sore throats.
— Sage: for sore throats, gargle with tea. Also use in com-press on the neck.

— Sytra tea (Weleda): for coughs, see instructions on the packet.

— WCS powder (Weleda): for small wounds and red spots, pat lightly on to the skin. Also use to treat a baby's navel.

— Cinabar pyrites tablets (Weleda): for a sore throat, take 2 tablets four times a day. Gargle regularly with sage tea.

— Bath thermometer and thermometer to take the patient's temperature

— sterile gauze and sterile plasters

— scissors

154

— vaseline

— safety pins

— various cloths in different sizes made of cotton, linen, flannel and wool for small compresses and body compresses.

It is important to store herbs in well-sealed jars. To prevent mistakes, it is advisable to label all bottles and tubes, and to note the date on which the contents were bought and used. Medicines should be stored in a cool, dark place, though not in the fridge unless specifically indicated.

Oils can no longer be used when they start to smell rancid. It is best to replace herbs with every new harvest. Most ointments, fluids and powders can be kept for a long time. However, after about three years their potency will be reduced. If you are unsure about the potency of a medicine because you have had it a long time, it is best to flush it down the toilet.

Endnotes

1. *Principles and Practice of Nursing,* p.14. Macmillan, New York, & Collier Macmillan, London, 6th ed. 1978.

2. Dr Ita Wegman, *Im Aufbruch des Wirkens für eine Erweiterung der Heilkunst.*

3. See Mees, *Secrets of the Skeleton,* SteinerBooks, 2005.

4. Examples may be found in *Prayers and Graces* collected by Michael Jones, or in *Meditative Prayers* by Adam Bittleston — both Floris Books, Edinburgh.

Index

acne 118
airing (of room) 54
arnica 67–69
art therapy 18, 30
asthma 122

back rest 55
bark 64
barley water 64
bath (therapeutic) 61
bed, making 53f
bed blocks 55
bed cradle 55
bedpan 48f
bed pull 55
bedside table 41
bedsores 56f
bed table 55
biography 23
birth 136
bladder, chill on 94f
bleeding, internal 68
boils 114, 118
bowel movement 45, 47
breast compress 116f
breast feeding 137
breathing 62
bronchitis 78, 102, 114, 122
bruising 68
bulking agents 47
burns 69, 71–73, 129, 153

calendula 83–85
camomile 85–95
carob oil 106
chest compress 78, 103
chicken pox 73
circulation 127
Clairo tea 47
cold 91f
combudoron 72
commode 49, 56
compress 61
—, arnica 67f
—, calendula 83–85
—, camomile 85–95
—, combudoron 72
—, curd cheese (quark) 114–18
—, horseradish 95–100
—, lemon 74–81
—, mustard 100–108
—, onion 109–113
—, stinging nettle 69–73
concussion 69
constipation 46f, 92–94
contractures 58
cradle 137f
cramp in calves 59
curd cheese 114–18

delirious 75
diarrhoea 47
drinking 45, 149

drop foot 58
dying 147–52

earache 110–13
enema 92–94
etheric body 25
etheric oils 34f, 106

fainting 60
fever 75
flower 35, 64
foot-bath 107f, 127–29
foot rest 55
fruit 63

headache 107f
herbal tea 63f
hives 72f
horseradish 95–100
hyperaemia 102

incontinence 50
inhalation 91f
insect bites 72f
insomnia 140f
internal bleeding 68

joints, inflammation of 110–13

last offices (undertaker's) 151
last rites (anointing) 150
lavender bath 124
lavender foot-bath 142

laxatives 47, 92
leaf (of plant) 35, 63f
lemon 74–81
light in sick room 41, 43

marigold 83–85
massage 61
mastitis 114, 116f
material for compress 62
meals 44
metabolic/limb system 28, 32
migraine 102
milk, milk products 45
mobilization 59
mouth, care of 45
mucous membrane irritation 102
mustard 100–108

nervous/sensory system 28, 32
nettle 69–73 (see also combudoron)
nutrition (during pregnancy) 134

oil bath 120–22
onion 109–13

pain killers 150
pneumonia 58, 102
potentizing 20
poultice 61, 129f
pregnancy 133–36

quark 114–18

rash (skin) 71–73

rest 46

rhythm 29

rhythmic system 29–33

root (of plant) 35, 63f

rosemary bath 124

rubber sheet 56

rubbing body 125–27

salt water wash 118f

seed 63f

senna pod tea 47

sentient (perceiving) soul 26

sheepskin fleece 56

sheets, changing 53f

shingles 72f

sinusitis 98

skin care 52

skin rash 71–73

skin tone lotion 52

sleep 139–43

sprains 69

stalk (of plant) 64

Steiner, Rudolf 7–9

stinging nettle 69–73

stomach-ache 91

stomach compress 90f

substance baths 122–24

sunburn 72f

swelling 68

tea, herbal 63–65

temperature of patient 50f

temperature of room 44

throat ache 81

throat compress 81

thrombosis 59

thyme oil 122

toothache 95

urination 46, 49

urine retention 59

urine bottle 50

ventilation (of room) 53f

vomiting 47

wash (therapeutic) 61

washing of patient 51–53

Wegman, Ita 9

wounds 83

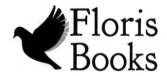

Floris Books

For news on all our **latest books,**
and to receive **exclusive discounts,**
join our mailing list at:

florisbooks.co.uk

Plus subscribers get a FREE book
with every online order!

We will never pass your details to anyone else.

www.ingramcontent.com/pod-product-compliance
Lightning Source LLC
Jackson TN
JSHW011352130125
77033JS00016B/568